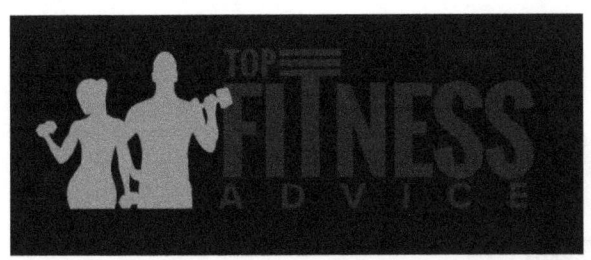

CALISTHENICS WORKOUT BIBLE

The #1 Guide For Beginners – Over 75+ Bodyweight Exercises (Photos Included)

Bruce Harlow

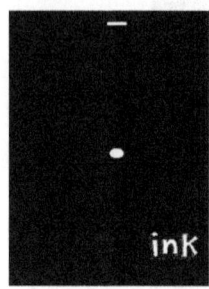

First published in 2017 by Venture Ink Publishing

Copyright © Top Fitness Advice 2019

All rights reserved.

No part of this book may be reproduced in any form without permission in writing from the author. No part of this publication may be reproduced or transmitted in any form or by any means, mechanic, electronic, photocopying, recording, by any storage or retrieval system, or transmitted by email without the permission in writing from the author and publisher.

Requests to the publisher for permission should be addressed to publishing@ventureink.co

For more information about the contents of this book or questions to the author, please contact Bruce Harlow at bruce@topfitnessadvice.com

Disclaimer

This book provides wellness management information in an informative and educational manner only, with information that is general in nature and that is not specific to you, the reader. The contents of this book are intended to assist you and other readers in your personal wellness efforts. Consult your physician regarding the applicability of any information provided in this book to you.

Nothing in this book should be construed as personal advice or diagnosis, and must not be used in this manner. The information provided about conditions is general in nature. This information does not cover all possible uses, actions, precautions, side-effects, or interactions of medicines, or medical procedures. The information in this book should not be considered as complete and does not cover all diseases, ailments, physical conditions, or their treatment.

You should consult with your physician before beginning any exercise, weight loss, or health care program. This book should not be used in place of a call or visit to a competent health-care professional. You should consult a health care professional before adopting any of the suggestions in this book or before drawing inferences from it.

Any decision regarding treatment and medication for your condition should be made with the advice and consultation of a qualified health care professional. If you have, or suspect you have, a health-care problem, then you should immediately contact a qualified health care professional for treatment.

No Warranties: The author and publisher don't guarantee or warrant the quality, accuracy, completeness, timeliness, appropriateness or suitability of the information in this book, or of any product or services referenced in this book.

The information in this book is provided on an "as is" basis and the author and publisher make no representations or warranties of any kind with respect to this information. This book may contain inaccuracies, typographical errors, or other errors.

Liability Disclaimer: The publisher, author, and other parties involved in the creation, production, provision of information, or delivery of this book specifically disclaim any responsibility, and shall not be held liable for any damages, claims, injuries, losses, liabilities, costs, or obligations including any direct, indirect, special, incidental, or consequences damages (collectively known as "Damages") whatsoever and howsoever caused, arising out of, or in connection with the use or misuse of the site and the information contained within it, whether such Damages arise in contract, tort, negligence, equity, statute law, or by way of other legal theory.

Table of Contents

Disclaimer	3
Introduction	7
The Advantages and Disadvantages of Calisthenics	9
Commitment and Goal Setting	17
Tips Before Starting	23
75+ Bodyweight Exercises	27
Conclusion	93
Final Words	95

Would you prefer to listen to my book, rather than read it?

Download the audiobook version for free!

If you go to the special link below and sign up to Audible as a new customer, you can get the audiobook version of my book completely free.

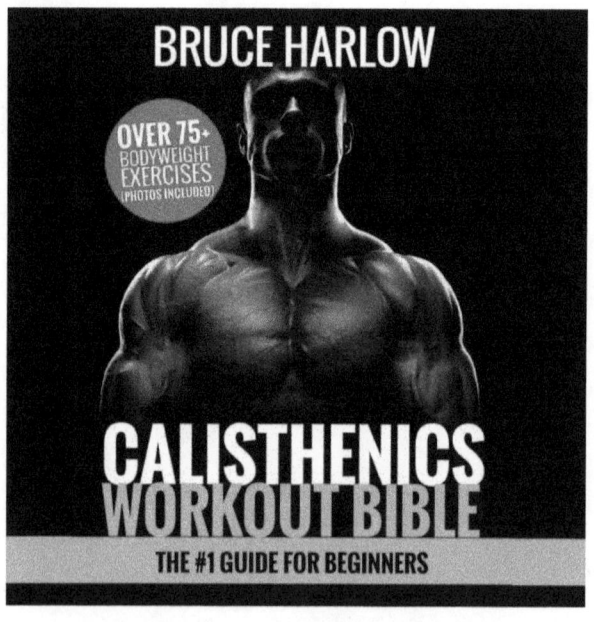

Go here to get your audiobook version for free:

TopFitnessAdvice.com/go/Calisthenics

Introduction

Finding the right exercise routine can be difficult. The routine you do choose depends on what you want to achieve. Calisthenics is a great routine if you want build strength through bodyweight exercises.

This book will focus on explaining what calisthenics is and what advantages and disadvantages as well as 75+ Bodyweight Exercises

What is it?

Calisthenics is derived from the Greek words 'kallos,' meaning beauty, and 'sthenos,' meaning strength, which points to calisthenics as a way of achieving beauty and strength.

It is as a way to develop physical fitness and beauty by using your own body weight. Generally, the exercises are carried without using any equipment. It is through mostly rhythmic movements that strength and flexibility are increased, using the body's own mass as resistance.

Jumps, bends, twists, swings and kicks are often done along with stretching exercises. When done regularly and energetically, calisthenics can improve cardiovascular and muscular strength, at the same time improving balance, coordination, and agility. This is why calisthenics is often the go-to exercise for military and sports teams, as well as part of school exercises in grade schools and high schools.

The Origins of Calisthenics

The ancient Greeks valued strength and physical fitness, as the legends of Hercules evince. They viewed the body as a temple for the soul and mind, something that needed to be kept healthy and optimal.

Calisthenics started out as gymnastics, where the body is tempered by progressive exercises that test agility, flexibility, and strength. Although calisthenics was dropped by the Greeks in favor of sports, calisthenics has become popular again.

Many favor calisthenics because of the ease with which you can start doing it; after all, you don't need much prior training or any special equipment. You don't even need a gym membership, just your own body and the determination to exercise.

Also, unlike most specialized muscle building routines, calisthenics works on you as a whole, improving strength, as well as flexibility and agility, as the ancient Greeks valued holistic learning above all else. This is why calisthenics holds a prominent place in free running circles, or parkour.

The Advantages and Disadvantages of Calisthenics

Advantages of Calisthenics

As mentioned above, calisthenics is a very old practice, and yet, is still relevant today. This only shows the effectivity and many benefits that can be derived from calisthenics. Below is a list of advantages that are clearly offered by calisthenics.

1. It can be learned with relative ease. In calisthenics, you don't really need to learn how to use special equipment and special routines. Since you're using your own body as a weight, you are relatively familiar with it.

   The resistance that you are using for your training is already fitted to your needs exactly. There are many beginners who find calisthenics easier to learn and do than using weights, such as barbells and dumbbells.

2. Relatively safe to do compared with other exercises. As you are only using your own body and not any special equipment, you are eliminating a lot of the risks. In calisthenics, you push your body within certain parameters, while the use of barbells and dumbbells allow beginners to add extreme amounts of weight that often leads to injury.

   Also, calisthenics requires you to progress through the exercises. You can't jump into the harder exercises on a whim. They cannot be done. You have to really work to be able to do the more challenging exercises. This means that your body is prepped for the next challenges. This is not true for other weight training procedures.

3. Calisthenics will benefit many athletic pursuits. The strength and agility you can gain in calisthenics also greatly affect your performance in a wide range of sports and athletics.

   There is no universally accepted theory as to why that is, but many believe that this is because calisthenics improves your physical fitness holistically.

4. The difficulty of the exercise is amped up by changing the muscles' capacity to exert force. Admittedly, this can be somewhat confusing.

   In calisthenics, since you are using your own bodyweight for resistance, you can't really add more body weight to make the exercises more challenging. What you can do is make it more challenging for your muscles to exert the effort by changing the position and manipulating the leverage of your muscles.

The Disadvantages of Calisthenics

1. It can be difficult building up great lower body strength. Since you are not using any weights as resistance, it can be very hard for you to develop lower body strength.

   As the biggest and most powerful muscles of the human body can be found in the lower body, such as the gluteus and quads, you also need a heck of a lot of resistance to achieve any considerable strength gains.

Of course, this can only become a concern if you are training specifically for lower body strength.

2. It is difficult to manipulate leverage and increase the resistance when it comes to the lower body. There really is no way around this fact.

   The lower body is just built in a way that does not allow for much leeway to design exercises with decreased leverage. This is basically why most calisthenics videos do not have much emphasis on lower body exercises.

3. The muscle mass you can build up is limited with calisthenics. Although this is still very much debated, it has become a popular opinion.

   Although you definitely CAN achieve great muscle mass and tone with calisthenics, there is some difference in the size and tone you can achieve if you do a lot of weight training.

   Again, calisthenics is more about building up your strength as a whole unit and not just to make certain muscles pop. If you want to have the muscle definition of a body builder, then it would be better if you did bodybuilding training.

4. The exercises you do can be limited as well. Although there are a lot of benefits with using your own body

weight as resistance, it is still true that this limits the exercises and training that you can do.

Your own body weight can only offer so much resistance. This means that exercises are limited to how much you can manipulate leverage, while the weight or resistance you put up can't really be altered.

Calisthenics is an age-old training and exercise regimen with its own set of advantages and disadvantages. Nevertheless, it is a great way to train your body to achieve feats that seem almost impossible and gain near superhuman strength.

I hope that you are enjoying this book so far, and if you could spare 30 seconds, I would greatly appreciate you leaving a review on Amazon.com.

Did You Know You Are MOST Likely Burning Fat Too SLOW?

Discover The Most POWERFUL Method to Start Burning Fat Up to 400% Faster!

For this month only, you can get Bruce's best-selling & most popular book absolutely free – *The Most Powerful Method to Burn Fat Up to 400% Faster!*

Get Your FREE Copy Here:
TopFitnessAdvice.com/Download

Discover exactly what you need to do to **put your metabolism into hyperdrive** and have your **fat melt away effortlessly**. And learn the biological "hacks" that have been scientifically proven to **boost the rate that your body burns fat by up to 400%.** With this book, readers were able to reach their fitness goals significantly quicker, so it's highly recommended that you get this book, especially while it's free!

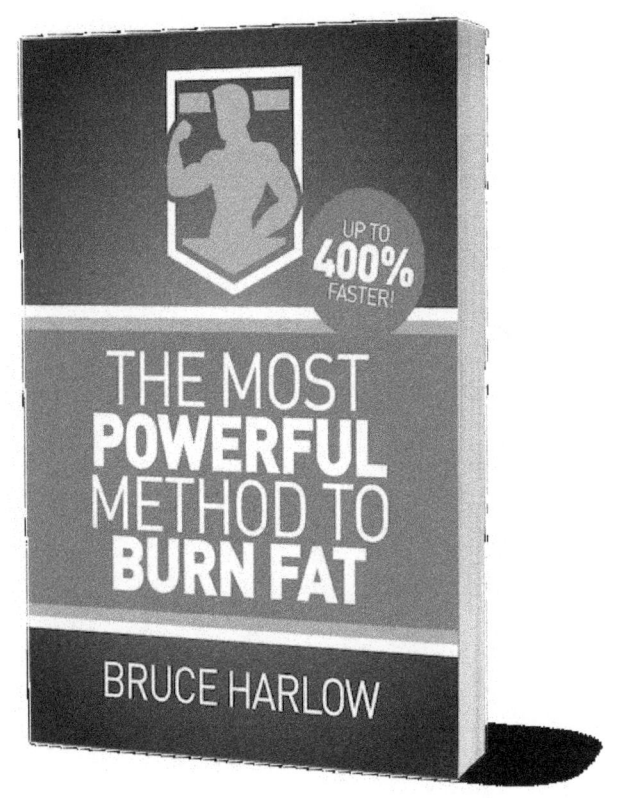

Get Your FREE Copy Here:

TopFitnessAdvice.com/Download

Commitment and Goal Setting

The magnificence of calisthenics works out is its utter independence! You can exercise anywhere, anytime, with an enormous diversity of movements and schedules. Isn't that fantastic?

It's extremely incredible if you know what you are accomplishing; however, if you're fresh to this kind of exercise or to any sort of exercise, then this may cause you to become puzzled. In particular for novices, it's important to have a well-thought-out routine to begin elaborating on a powerful foundation.

Set Your Objectives

Objectives are an imperative component of calisthenics. You need to be very logical about your objectives such as weight reduction, achievement of power, enhancement of muscle mass, upgrading of general health and stamina, achieving the skill to perform a precise work out such as the human flag.

Diverse objectives will call for different lines of attack. It is essential to make out what precisely you desire to do, for the reason that different objectives necessitate different approaches in how you exercise.

How to Commence?

This is a weighty question!

Well! Like the whole lot in life, begin with the fundamentals; before behaving in a playful way with difficult workouts such as front lever, planche and human flags.

Go off to the floor to perform a few push-ups, simple isn't it? Don't search for shorter alternative routes as it requires a certain period of time to convert your being into a muscle machine. However, it is mandatory for you to constantly place objectives happening in a relatively short period of time, so as to keep you energized.

Instead of making it a short-term obligation, coerce yourself to make it a way of everyday life! Furthermore, you have to be brilliant at the nitty-gritty such as:

- **Different pull-ups**: This exercise is necessary to reinforce your V-shape and upper limbs, along with subordinate muscles like your abdominal muscles as well as those of your shoulders.

- **Pushups**: This exercise will construct your sturdy chest and triceps, and subordinate muscles such as those of your shoulders.

- **Squats**: This exercise is meant to build up your legs

- **Diverse dips**: This exercise is accountable for building up the part of the entire body above the waist.

- **Abdominal exercises**: These are meant to give you a sturdy central part which is essential for calisthenics.

- **Leg raises**: This is the ideal exercise for the rather overlooked lower abdominal muscles as well as the flexors of your hips (the iliopsoas.) Carrying out leg raises frequently can facilitate to give a boost to your lower back and consequently decrease the possibility of injury.

Each and every advanced and more difficult movement is simply an adaptation or mishmash of these fundamental workouts. So you need to be very steady in those fundamental composite workouts so as to put up power inside you.

How to Make Headway in Calisthenics Successfully?

There are quite a few rules of development that you have to be aware of. On the whole, any expertise can be realized simply by becoming acquainted with these ethics.

Deconstruction

It simply means devoting a significant amount of your time to learn the expertise and dealing with it right from the start to the final result. In the case of calisthenics, you will have to put into practice the hollow body position. This is meant to fortify your principal muscles; so what you could do is to perform the following to a large extent:

- Intense squatting
- Dead lifting
- Kettle bells

- Swings and snatches
- Sandbag squats
- Shouldering

If you reject putting in weights to your exercise routine, there is a chance that you might be powerless to construct an amazing lower back. Anyways, you need to focus on concave body position, handstands and bridges.

Continuous Confrontation

Keep practicing and persevering as a habit. Challenge yourself by increasing difficulty constantly. Though it may be not so easy, yet with repeated attempts you will become more skillful in this.

Steadiness

According to the American football coach and player Vince Lombardi, "Practice does not make perfect. Only perfect practice makes perfect."

So you see! There is no shortcut to tough work, hard practice and determination; it is said that to become excellent at anything you need ten thousand hours of run through. As a matter of fact, you don't merely need a bit of practice, but sufficient and successful practice.

Tolerance and steadiness on your part will carry positive outcomes for you. Even if you possess quite good knowledge regarding the expertise and you may be making the finest headway, yet without faultless repeated attempts, all that is only speculation. Some guidelines to keep you steady are as follows:

- Lay down sensible targets that embrace obvious high points, and as you move forward toward your targets, you'll discover a ripple effect happens and things begin to make sense in your job, domestic routine, and physical condition.

- Put a uniform workout time on your calendar; this is the usual practice approved by some of the most dedicated exercisers; most of them perform it on a daily basis before sunrise or nocturnally.

- If you want to be more honest to your body, take an extra initiative with your daily calendar and attempt to foster thirty minutes every day; as a result, you will have more vigor and can be more well-organized.

  Then you'll find you have more energy and can be more efficient throughout the day. You may also make use of the cell phone tools such as e-mail mementoes on a day to day basis, workout chronicle websites as well as apps to keep you on task.

- Maintain a work out journal which should pursue your advancement; not only will it encourage you to make efforts but it will also assist you, to decide how to take any further steps forward.

- Keep track of your advancement by keeping records of every one minor accomplishment. Targets, regarding something you want to do in the near future are trouble-free to maintain, and every miniature accomplishment will assist to keep encouraged.

- Do record your opinion after every calisthenics workout, so that when you are at a low level on enthusiasm to rise from sleep and go for an exercise, you can withdraw it and glance at the feelings jotted down by you after doing the calisthenics workout successfully. This will truly make you appreciate that at the closing stages of the workout, you will experience the same wonderful feeling again.

- Perform a bit of miniscule workout on a daily basis so as to assist you keep up the routine of exercises all through the week.

    These miniscule workouts may consist of core movements, usual pushups and hang-ups.) Your core will perform as a counterbalance and hub. As a consequence, when your real training days will arrive, a much smaller amount of your exertion will be spent.

Once again, thank you for reading this book, and I hope you're getting a lot of valuable information. I would greatly appreciate it if you could take 30 seconds to leave me a review for this book on Amazon.com.

Tips Before Starting

We may have convinced you to try out calisthenics, but before you do anything else, keep in mind that you should never do calisthenics halfheartedly. You should prepare both your mind and body before attempting any of the exercises that you will see on the internet.

Remember that even though calisthenics will lessen your chance of getting an injury, but if you attempt to do a high-level callisthenic exercise without prior experience and the proper body strength and stamina, then you are just waiting for a disaster to happen.

The most common mistake that beginners usually commit when attempting to do calisthenics is that the exercise routines that they do are not done properly.

There are a lot of cases where in people would give up doing exercises or workouts after a few months because they fail to see the results of their hard work. It may be because the results needed at least a couple more months to show the progress, as most people would assume, but that is rarely the case. The main reason for their failure is that they are doing the exercises wrong.

You will only just tire yourself by doing 50 incorrect pushups. No matter how many push up or sit-ups you do, if you are doing it incorrectly then you are just wasting your time and effort. It is better to do just 5 push-ups, done properly, rather than doing 20 incorrect ones.

Remember that it is essential that you control your muscular motions when doing these exercises, you will not be able to build the muscles that you want if you are fooling yourself in performing incorrect exercises.

Try to do simple calisthenics routines first. We will discuss in another chapter a set of simple exercises that you could try out for yourself. Try to repeat these simple exercises and increase the sets little by little. Take note of your progress.

If you feel that you've improved, try to raise the level of difficulty gradually. If you feel that a certain part of your body needs more work, they include exercises in your workout routine that will strengthen that specific part.

Also, keep in mind that your desired body will not show up the next day after you just started your exercise. Getting your desired results may take some time.

Do not give up that easily when you fail to see your progress after a few days. Patience will reap rewards. The people that you see on the internet performing perfect calisthenics routines have years of training under their belt.

If you are doing calisthenics because you want to lose weight, then you should incorporate diet in your meals and to not just rely on callisthenic exercises to shed that extra pounds.

Calisthenics aims to build your muscles and body strength. Although it could be an effective way to lose weight, but exercising alone will not do the trick.

You yourself should discover the wonders of calisthenics and what it could do to you and your body. Keep your motivation up by watching videos on calisthenics and reading related material.

75+ Bodyweight Exercises

Lower Body Exercises

There are different yoga poses and techniques used for many centuries to get health benefits. If you don't have a couple of hours to attend the yoga classes, there is no need to worry because you can select some of your favorite yoga postures to feel the incredible power of yoga postures.

Following are some yoga postures and poses with a detailed explanation to follow them:

1. Malasana (Yoga Squat)

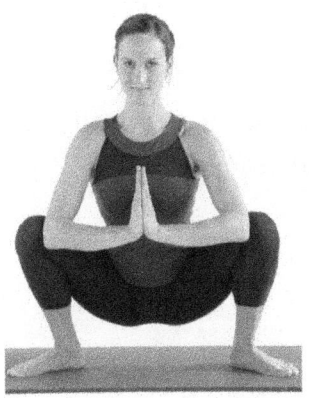

The Malasana is a famous squatting yoga posture with toes out and the heels in. Sit in with toes out and heels in with the hands in the prayer position in front of your chest. The posture is perfect for pregnant ladies get relief of backache and stretch the calves and inner thighs.

2. Half Moon

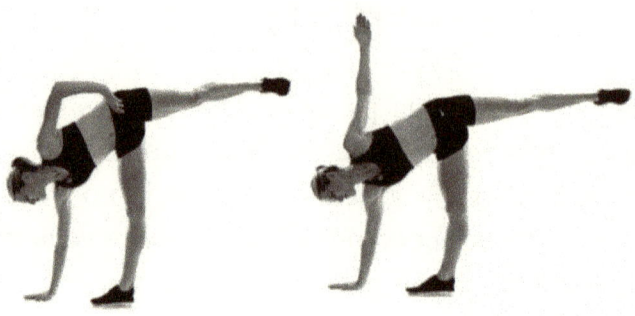

The posture is good for the brain and nervous system because you have to make a balancing pose light up your mind. Balance your right leg and right hand while lifting the left leg in the parallel position to the floor.

The left arm will be extended in the straight position. It is an important posture because you can challenge your body to maintain a balance to gracefully handle signs of aging.

3. Gratitude Meditation

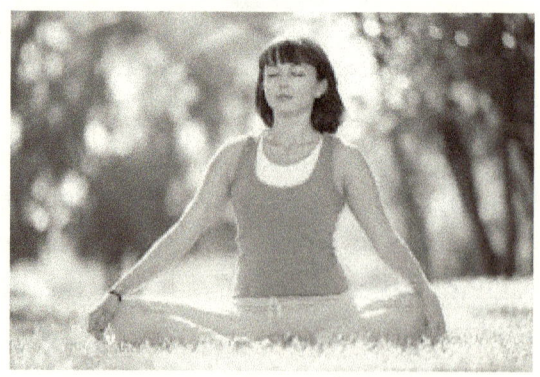

It is a common form of meditation in which you can bring some positive energy in your body by thinking about the comforts and luxuries you have in your life. Feel grateful for everything to get rid of depression and anxiety.

4. Nostril Breathing

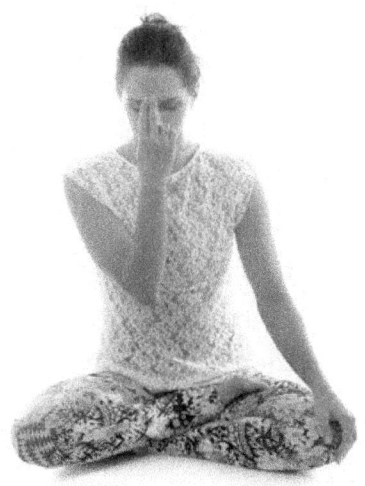

A form of yogic breathing from alternate nostrils will help you to release stress and anxiety. Sit in the comfortable position and breathe from both nostrils, one by one to get equilibrium of the autonomic nervous system. It is a great posture to clean your lymphatic system.

5. Camel Pose

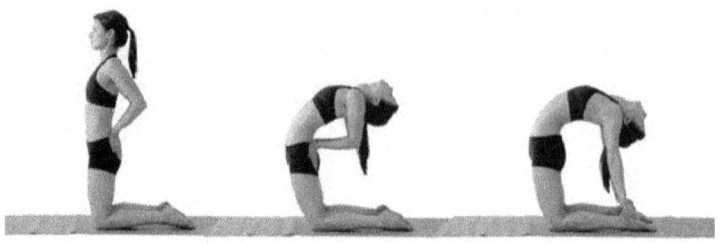

A great pose to increase the capacity of your lungs, stimulate the functions of the thyroid, pituitary and thyroid glands. The pose is really easy:

Stand on your knees with and place your hands on the hips. The tops of your feet should be placed on the mat. Bend in the backward direction while holding your heels to lengthen your spine. Stretch your neck and curl your head in the backward direction. Move your hands to the soles of your feet just for ten seconds.

6. Bound Angle

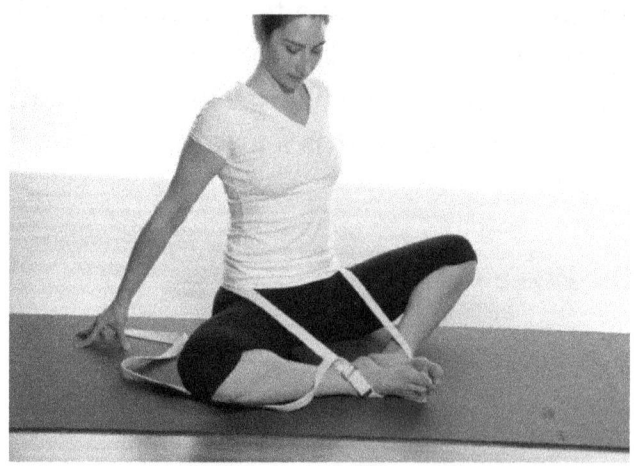

The bound angle is a useful, but simple yoga posture to gently open your hips and shoulders to relieve the symptoms of the menstrual cycle in women, menopause and other disorders of pelvic organs. The pose is really easy to follow:

Just sit on the floor and join the soles of both feet together while keeping the knees toward the floor.

Stack your shoulders to hips, but you can also bend in the forward direction, or prefer to sit straight. Inhale and exhale in the similar position for almost 4 to 8 times.

7. Warrior 1

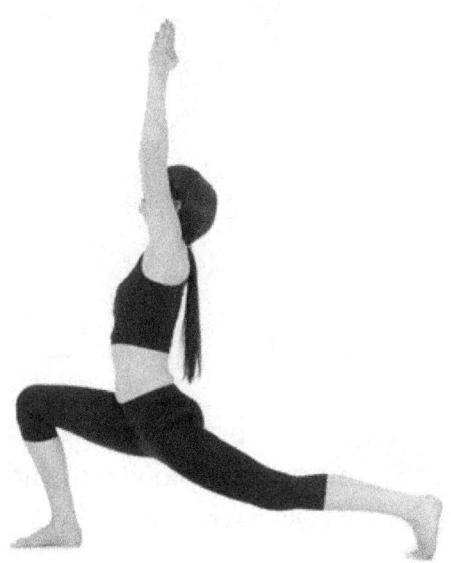

The posture is perfect to stretch main abdominal muscle called the Psoas. The Psoas tension can be experienced in the body through jaws, mouth tension and grinding of the teeth. The pose will help you to release overall tension of your body. To practice this posture:

Stand on your feet by keeping them almost 4.5 feet apart with front toes in the forward position and back foot on a slight angle.

Keep the front knee parallel to the front ankle, and the thigh should be placed parallel to the floor. The arms should be extended to the head while keeping the shoulder, chest and hips to quadrangle forward to the front of the room.

8. Wheel of Vitality

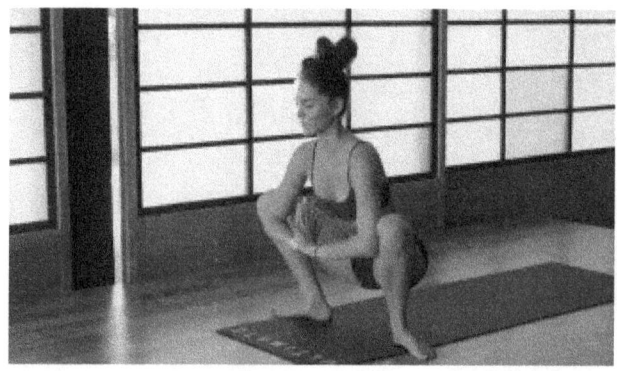

The posture is perfect for the better health of the cardiovascular system, and you can improve the blood circulation in your body. You can repeat this posture several times to get its benefits.

Stand on your feet while keeping them wide apart with heels in the inward and the toes in the outer direction. Bend the knees toward toes and squats toward floor to maintain the aligned position of knees.

Bend the hands toward heart and start tai-chi type movements, such as, open the arms and bring the hands together in the heart. Pressed the hands toward the sky and then bring them back to the floor. Sweep your hands down to the foot and make a big circle in the forward direction.

Reverse the hands circular movements in the opposite direction and repeat the movements of arm three times to get steady squat.

9. Half Lord of the Fishes Pose

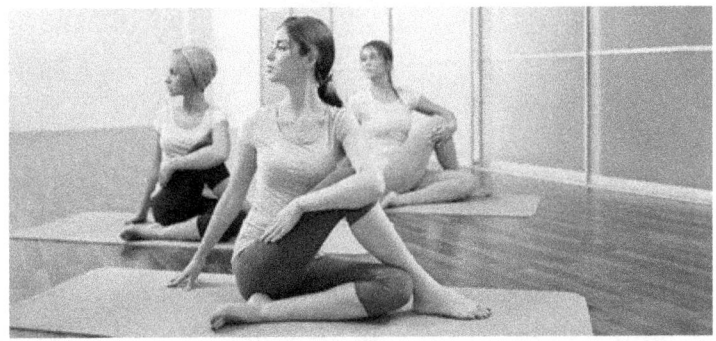

The pose is perfect to improve the digestive system and organs. It helps you to reduce back pain by unwinding the muscles of the lower back. The posture is really easy to follow:

Sit on the floor with straight legs in front of you. Bend the left knee and put your feet on the floor. Cross the right foot on the top and stick your knee in the straight direction.

Support your body by keeping the right hand on the floor behind you. Bend the left elbow and place it on the right thigh to form a twist.

Repeat the movement to the other side and try to twist to the maximum spinal length. This will be a good pose to improve your digestive system and lower back pain.

10. Forearm Plank

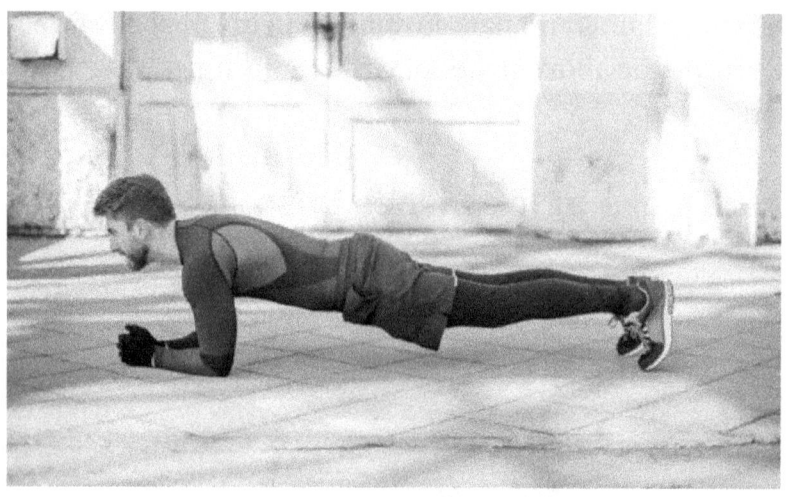

The posture will help you to increase the strength of your body and skeletal system to prevent osteoporosis. The posture is quite easy to follow, such as:

It is quite similar to the push-up, so lay your body in the push-up position, but hold your body on your forearms. Keep the shoulders and palm flat on the floor and the back of your toes will be tucked to keep the body in the line of energy.

You will get energy from the crown to the heels due to this posture. It is an excellent posture for students to give strength to the skeleton of your body.

11. Squat Jumps

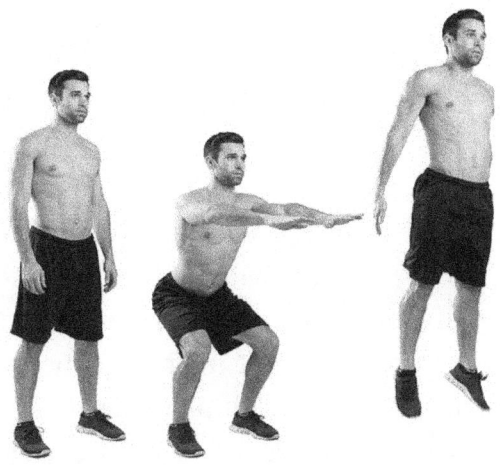

(Targeted muscle groups: Gluts and Thighs) This exercise starts out the same as a traditional squat, but when you reach the lowest point of your squat, you want to use your legs to push up forcefully, causing you to jump up. Reach above your head with outstretched arms to engage your whole body.

12. Lunges

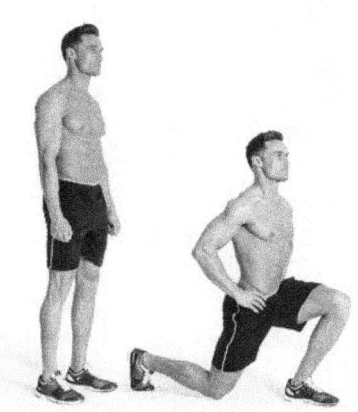

(Targeted muscle groups: Gluts and Thighs) To get into proper position for a lunge, start in a standing position and step forward with one leg. (The exact distance you need to go depends on the length of your leg, so you will have to adjust the distance initially so that you can execute the movement correctly.)

Be sure to put most of your weight on your forward foot and keep yourself mostly upright with a slight lean forward. Then bend the knee of your back leg and lower your hips down towards the floor until your knee nearly touches and then push back up to starting position. Complete repetitions on one leg, then switch to the opposite leg and repeat the exercise.

13. Walking Lunges

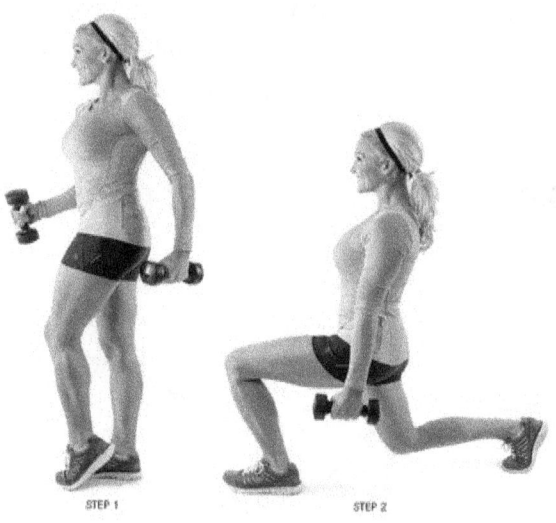

(Targeted muscle groups: Gluts and Thighs) This is a variation of the traditional lunge. In this exercise, start by stepping forward, lowering the knee on your rear leg down to the floor, and as you push back up to a standing position, bring your rear leg forward to take another step.

This will leave your opposite leg behind you to lower down, push back up and then step forward. Each lunge counts as one repetition.

Step Up: (Targeted muscle groups: Gluts, Thighs, and Calf) One of the simplest exercises to do is a stair climb or step up. You can use a traditional staircase or increase the distance to step up by using a street curb, a step stool, or a sturdy chair.

You will want to keep your hips and shoulders in alignment, back straight, and abs engaged, and then use one leg to step up and back down. Then repeat with opposite leg to complete one repetition.

14. Calf Raises

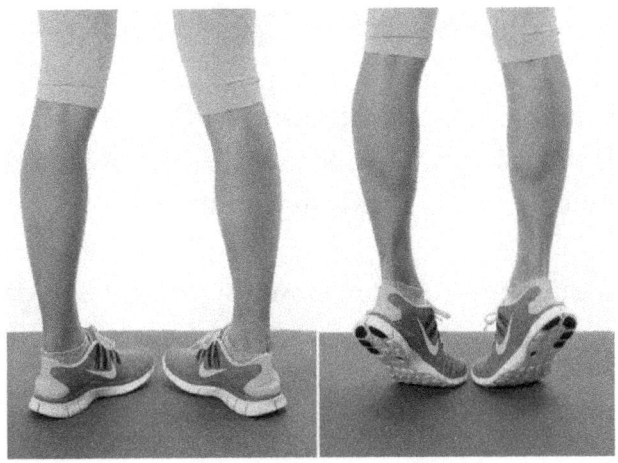

(Targeted muscle groups: Calf) For this exercise, it is helpful, at least at first, to have a chair or railing to help steady keep your body steady. Using a step or box, stand only on the front of your feet leaving the arch back to the heels off the edge.

Then press up on your toes, engaging your calf muscles and raising up your body as if wearing heels. Slowly lower back down to your starting position to complete and repeat.

15. Calf Lowers

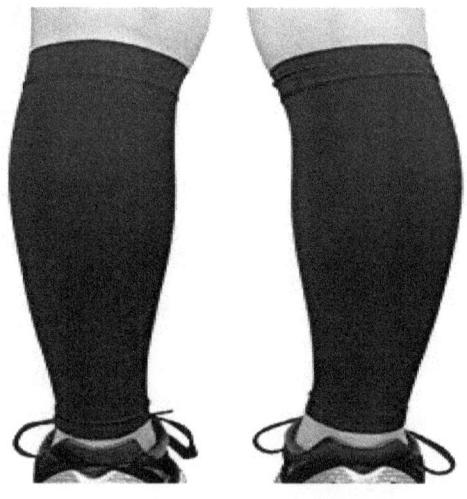

(Targeted muscle groups: Anterior Calf) This is the opposite exercise to calf raises and works a little bit more of the muscles on the front of your leg, opposite your calves.

Starting in the same position, slowly dip your heels down ward and then push back up. This is a good exercise to couple with the raises in order to work opposite muscle groups.

16. Sumo Squat

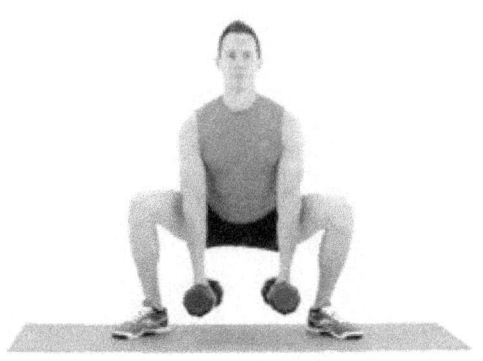

(Targeted muscle groups: Inside and Outside Thighs) For this squat variation, you simply want to change your stance. Move your feet slightly wider than shoulder width apart, place your hands on your knees for added stability, and perform the traditional squat motion. Press down and push up for one repetition.

17. Wall Sit

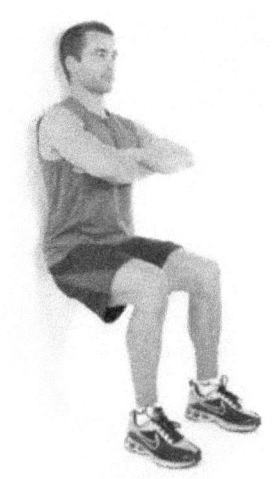

(Targeted muscle groups: Thighs) This exercise is performed exactly as the name describes. You want to simply put yourself into a seated position while pressing your back against a wall.

As you progress through these exercises, it will become apparent that some are becoming too easy so simply increase repetitions or add an additional set. In order to maintain intensity and continue to see results, it may be time to increase the difficulty of the movement rather than just repeating the same motion until you lose count. So, how do you up the ante and achieve the increased difficulty?

Keep in mind that progressing to the next level of an exercise is completely individualized. So, there is no one person that can tell you when it is time to move up to the next level for any one move; however, if you add in one or two reps of a new variation to your current workout, it can eventually replace the exercise you are currently doing.

You will also find that it may be a bit easier to increase the intensity this way rather than trying to pull off a much harder movement. Now, it is time to look at some advanced moves.

Enjoying this book?

Check out our other best sellers!

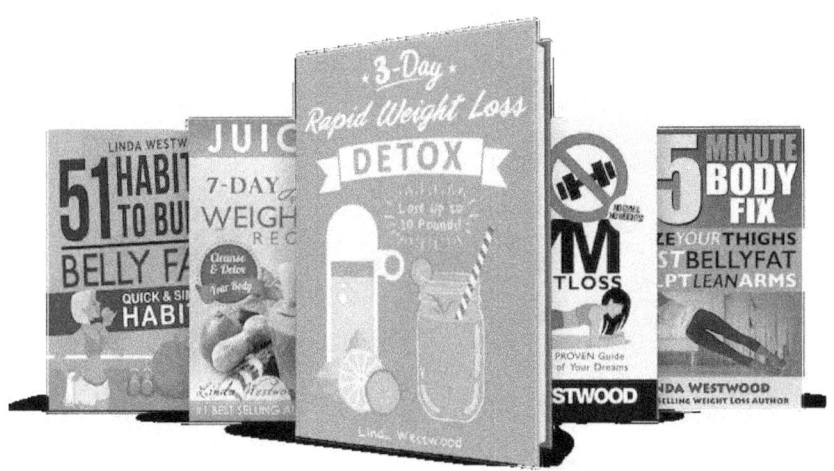

Get your next book on sale here:

TopFitnessAdvice.com/go/books

Standards Push-Ups, Lunges, And Stretches

There are few exercises that proves helpful to reduce a good amount of weight. You can follow these exercises:

18. Pushups with Alterations

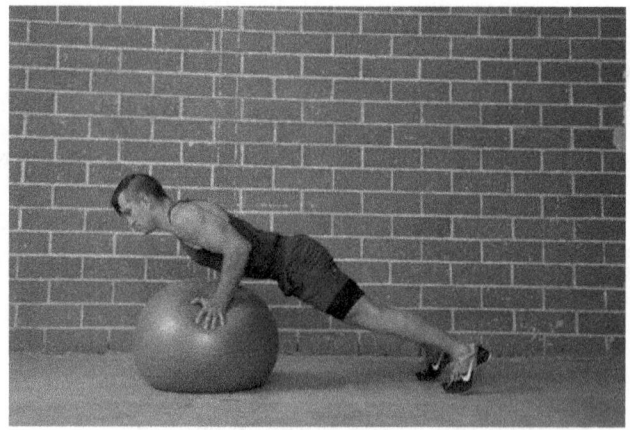

Push-ups are great movements to reduce overall body fat and keep rotating your one arm off the floor. Your head should follow the moving arm and it is important to maintain control and lower your arm in the pushup position. See the image above to know more about this position.

19. Spiderman Lunges

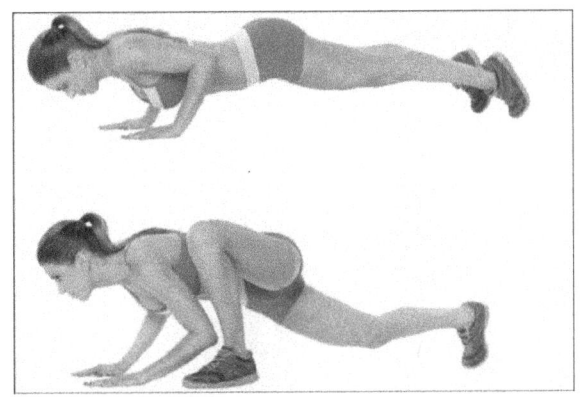

It is just like pushups, but you have to set the posture of your body before doing it. Above given image will help you to understand the actual posture.

20. Up-down Plank

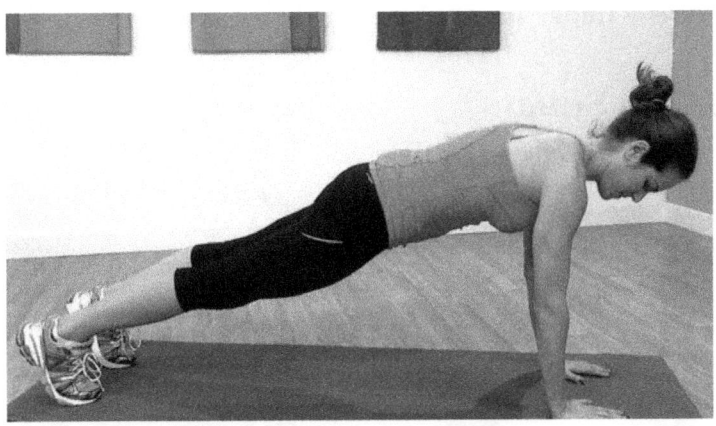

Set a modified plank position on your forearms while keeping your palm on the floor. Keep your left hand inside under your shoulders and press down your body up. Walk your other hand, in a plank position with the straight arm. See the above give picture to practice this position.

21. Lateral Lunges

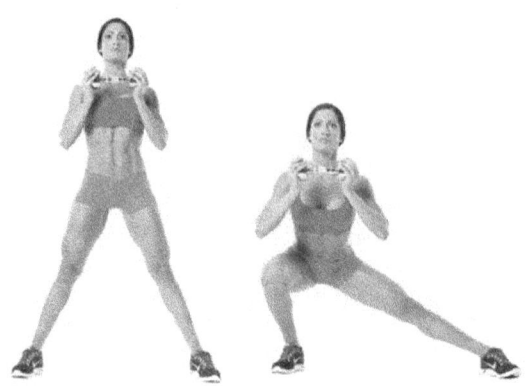

Start it by standing on your feet with hands on hips and step out the right while shifting your body weight from the right leg to form 90-degree angle and then shift it to the left leg in a similar way. See the image above.

22. Jump Squats

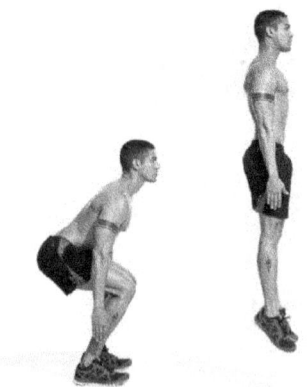

Cross your arms on the chest and keep your head up with a straight back. Set your feet at the shoulder width and keep your back straight and squat down while you inhale. Keep your upper thighs parallel to the flower. Exert force at the balls of your feet and jump up in the air as high as possible. Your thighs will play the role of spring. See the image above.

23. Mountain Climbers

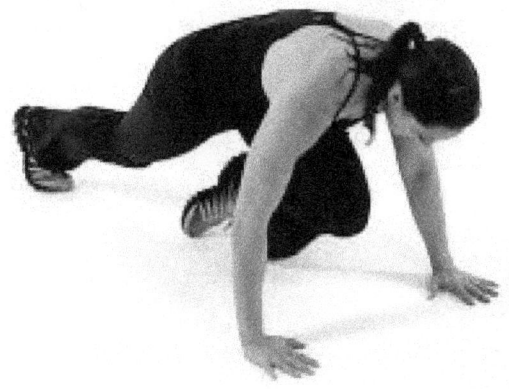

It is a full body workout and numerous muscles may work on this exercise, such as biceps, triceps, oblique, lower trapezius, quadriceps, hip, hamstrings, etc.

Start this with pushup position, and your weight will be supported by your hands and toes.

Flex the knee and hips and bring one leg to an approximate position. This will be a starting position, now explosively reverse your legs at the same position. See the image above.

24. Bodyweight Sit Through

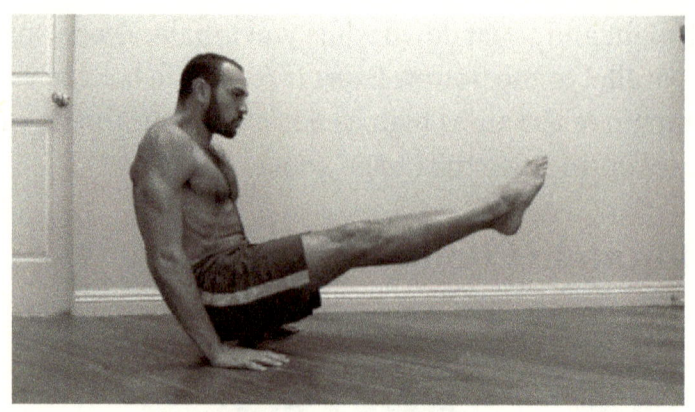

Start with your hands and knees and rise up on your toes and make your core firm. Rotate your body by moving your left hand up to your chest and ps your leg through the available space under your body. You can reverse these moves as per as you feel comfortable. You can rotate your both legs, one by one, and given above picture will give you an idea of this exercise:

25. Ice Skaters

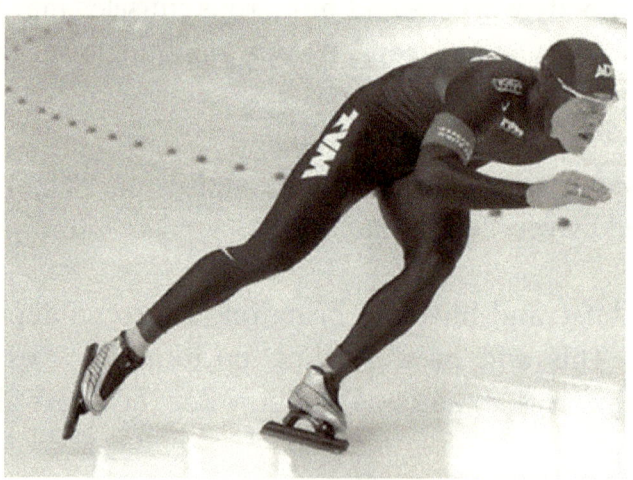

Start this exercise by standing on one leg and hop from side to side. Switch your legs while hoping and swing your arms while touching opposite legs. See the above image.

26. Prone Cobra

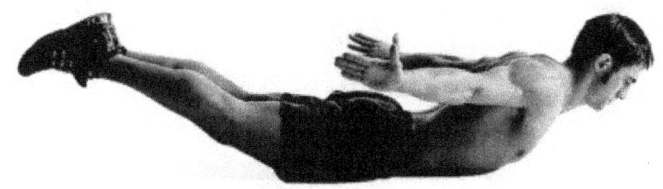

It is an endurance exercise that enables you to make your belly flat. Just lie down while keeping your belly horizontal on the floor. Spread your hands on the floor while lying on the floor. Above image will help you to understand the posture.

27. Skinny Dip

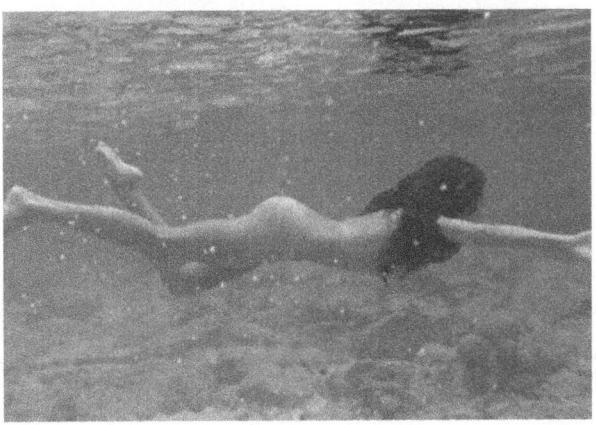

It is a great exercise for abs and it is really simple to do at your house. To do this exercise, you need to lie down on the floor on the left side and proper up your left arm and bend your knees at a 90-degree angle.

Lift the hip off the floor and raise the bent right leg almost a few feet. You can repeat this move for the both sides, and the above-given picture will be helpful.

28. Stretches for Standing Side

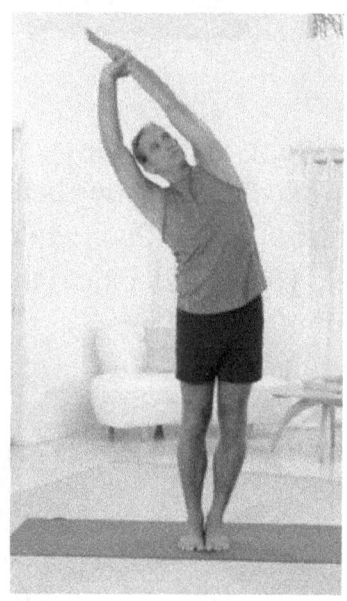

You have to stand on your feet together and keep your arms straight on your head. You should join your hands together while keeping your fingers interweaved and pointed. Inhale after reaching the upward position and exhale as you bend your upper body to the right and left. It is a good exercise to reduce the fat from your love handles.

29. Forward Hang

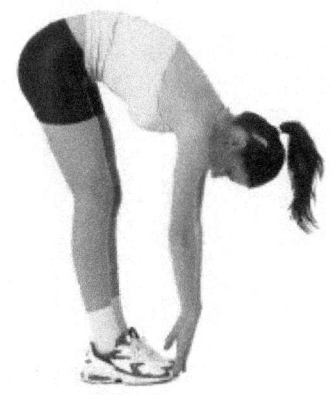

Stand straight on your feet while keeping the knees slightly bend. Join your fingers at the back of your back or if it is difficult to hold hands, you can carry a dish in both hands. Inhale; inflate your chest as you straighten your arms to chest.

Now exhale and bend at your waist while stretching your hand and exhale. It will be good to maintain this position for five seconds and take deep breaths.

30. Lunge Arch

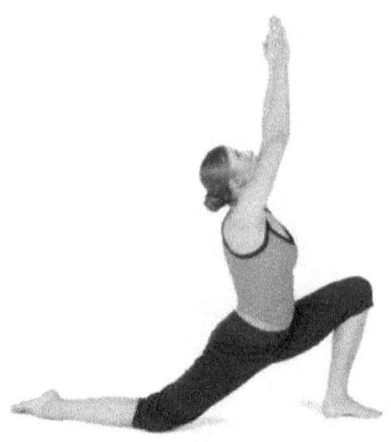

Keep your right foot onward into a lunge position and lower the position of left knee on the floor. You can keep a folded towel under your knee and bring both arms in the front position of your right leg. It will be good to hook both thumbs while keeping the palm towards the floor.

Inhale as you sweep the arms on the head and stretch to a comfortable position. Take deep breaths 5 to 10 times before switching.

Others who are considering purchasing this book would love to know what you think. If you could spare a few seconds, they would greatly appreciate reading an honest review from you. Simply visit the page on Amazon.com.

Dips, Raises and Lunges

The next exercises contained in this section will work your entire body, particularly building up your arms and your legs. They include the following:

31. Chest Dips on a Straight Bar

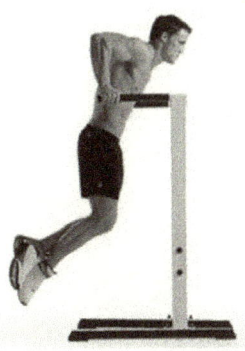

This exercise is excellent for building your upper body and will help to strengthen your triceps, anterior deltoids and pectorals. It can easily be done between two chairs if you do not have the straight bars where you work out.

You should begin by grabbing hold of the dip bars, and jump up. Ensure that your arms are straight and bend your knees gently. Slowly lower your body until your shoulders are lower than your elbows. Lean forward to maintain your balance.

32. Bench Dips

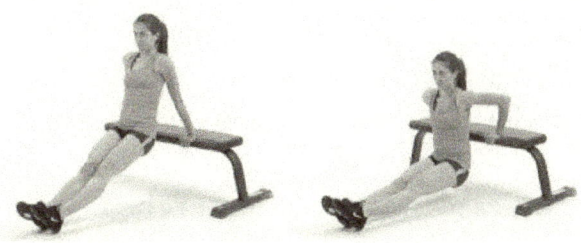

This is a great way to start building up your triceps. Place your feet on one bench and balance your upper body using the other bench. Keeping your arms rigid, bend them at the elbows and slowly lower your body to a 90-degree angle. Hold the position for several seconds and the get back into the starting position.

33. Dip to Leg Raisers

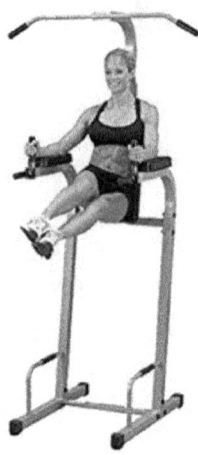

This exercise may seem simple but is much harder to execute than it seems. To execute a Dip to Leg raiser, first grab hold of either parallel dip bars or two chairs, and perform a standard dip.

However, when you are raising yourself up, begin to swing your legs forward so that when you are at the top of the motion your legs are stretched out in front of you. Hold the position for a few seconds, then lower your legs to complete the exercise.

This exercise is especially good for your chest and abs.

34. Incline Dip

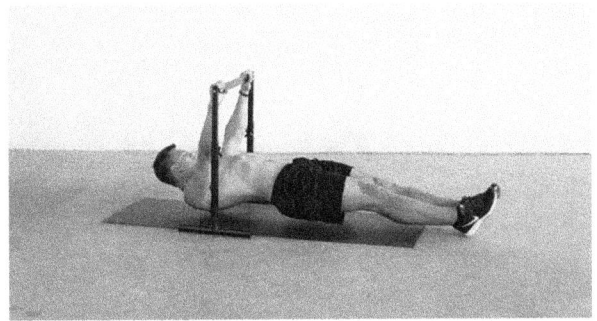

The Incline dip is a very good exercise for building your chest and triceps while reducing the risk of inuring your shoulders.

To execute an Incline Dip, hold the parallel bars and lift yourself off the ground. While doing so, raise your knees towards your chest so that your thighs are parallel to the ground (like you are sitting in a chair). You will need to hold them at this angle for the rest of the exercise.

Lower yourself down until your upper arms are parallel to the ground and your elbows have bent 90°, allowing your upper body to swing forward to maintain balance. Hold this position for a few seconds then return to the starting position.

35. One Arm Triceps Dips

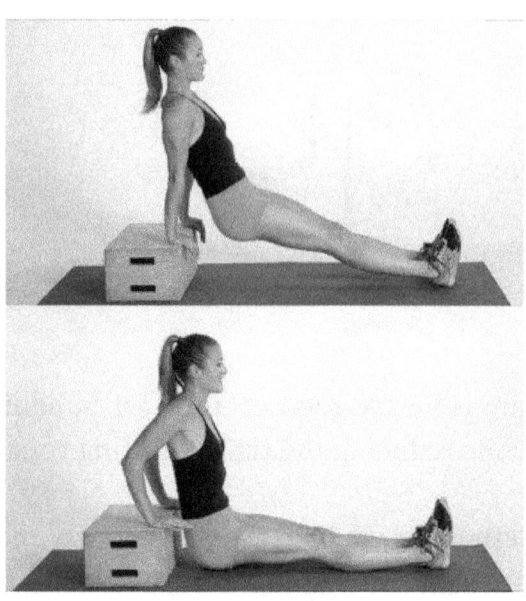

This is a more challenging variation to the standard dip. To perform this exercise, first enter the classic dip position, with your arms on a bench or a chair supporting your body in a sitting position.

Then, lift your right arm and left leg so that they are parallel with the ground, and you are only resting on your left arm and right leg. From this position, lower yourself until your elbow is at a 90° angle, keeping your extended arm and leg straight in the process.

Raise yourself back up to complete the exercise, and switch to the opposite position at the end of the set. If you would like to challenge yourself, you could switch legs after every rep, almost like a Russian Cossack dancer. This should help exercise your abs as well.

36. Leg Raises

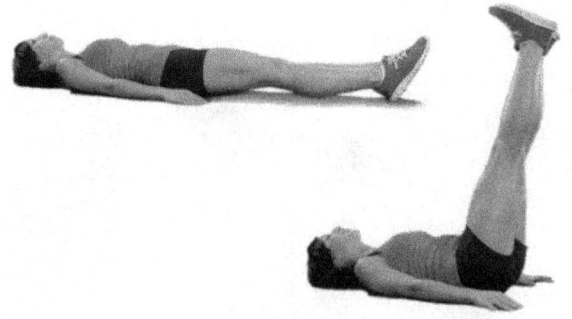

Start by hanging straight from a pull up bar. Raise your legs until they are at a 90-degree angle at the waist. Try to push your abdominal muscles towards your spine. Hold in position for a few seconds then slowly go back to the starting point.

37. Lying Leg Raises

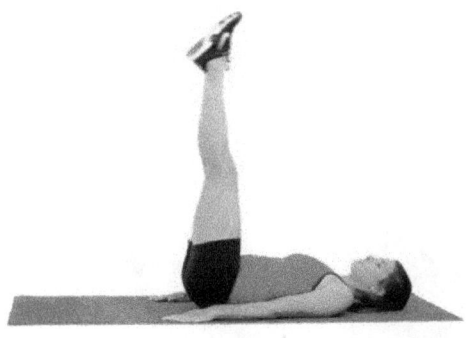

Lie down with your back straight and legs straight. Keep your hands on the sides, holding the bench. This is the starting position. Raise your legs slowly until they make a 90-degree angle from the waist. Keep your knees straight. Hold that position then slowly return to the starting position.

38. Lying Torso Raises

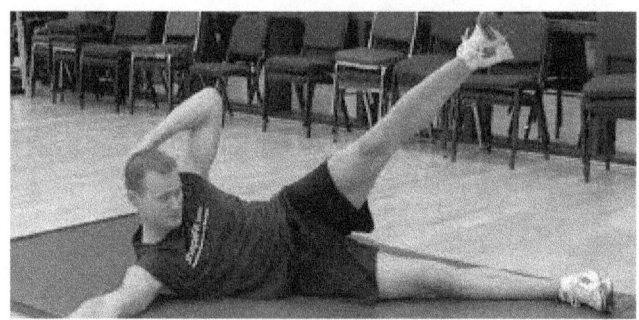

Lie on the floor, with your face down. Loosely place your hands on your sides with your palms facing down. This is the starting position. Slowly raise your torso until your chest is off the ground and then extend your neck back as you look at the ceiling. This should contract your lower back muscles. Hold for a few seconds, then slowly go back in the starting position.

39. Lying Side Leg Raises

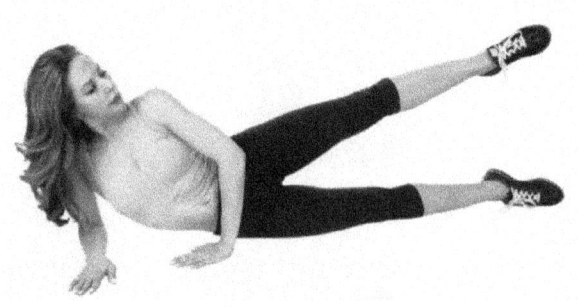

Begin this exercise by lying down on your side. Use one arm to support your head and place the other arm, palm down in front of you. Extend both eggs out keeping the straight.

Lift one leg up towards the ceiling keeping your toes pointed until you reach a 90-degree angle. Repeat several times. Turn and repeat on the other side.

40. Side Leg Raises

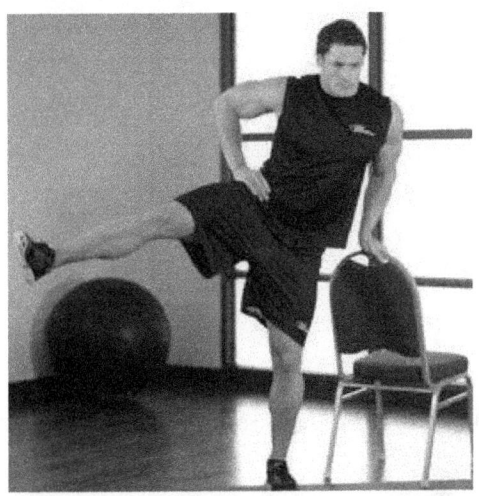

Lie down on your side for the starting position. Place your head on your arm, keeping it folded so that your head rests on the crook near your elbow.

Keep the other hand placed on the ground, palm down. Your legs should be straight. Slowly raise your leg up until you reach a 60-degree angle. Hold, and then lower it down. Repeat on the other side.

41. Straight Leg Raise

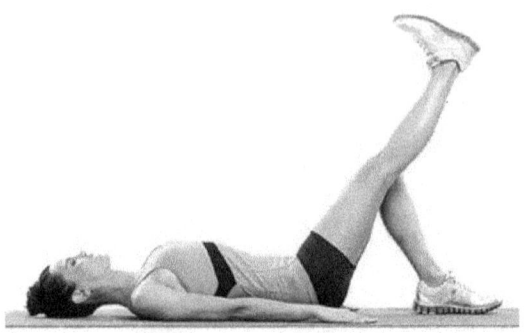

Start this exercise by lying down flat on yoour back. You should place a rolled towel under your neck for support. Keep your arms straight at your sides. Without bending your knees, lift one leg until you can see your toes. Hold for a moment and lower. Repeat with the other leg.

42. Glute/Hamstring Raises

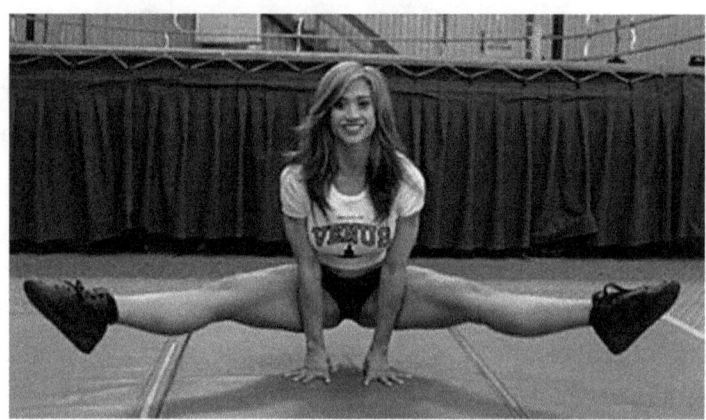

To perform this exercise, you will need a partner or somewhere you can brace your feet. Begin by getting onto your knees, keeping your upper legs and upper body upright.

Lower your body by leaning forward, making sure that you keep your body straight and restrict hip movement. Put your hands in front of you as you near the bottom of the movement, and slowly push yourself off the floor to help you return to the start position.

43. Squatted Calf Raises

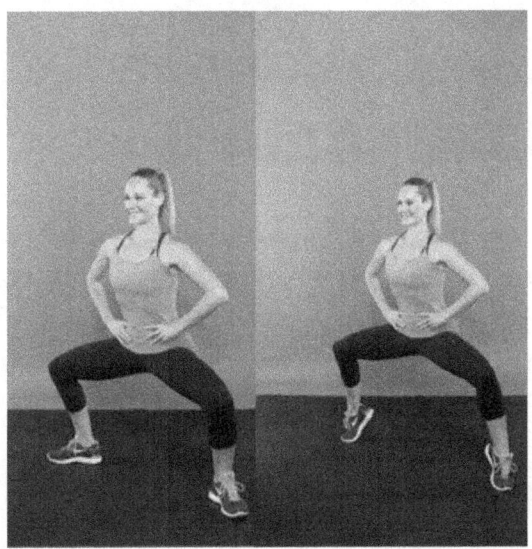

This is another interesting variation to a popular exercise that targets your whole lower body, from your glutes to your calves. To perform this exercise, lower yourself into the standard squatting position, then, while keeping your back straight, lift your heels until you are standing on your toes.

Hold the position for a few seconds, then return to the squatting position. Remember not to return to the standing position until you have completed one set.

44. Dragon Flag

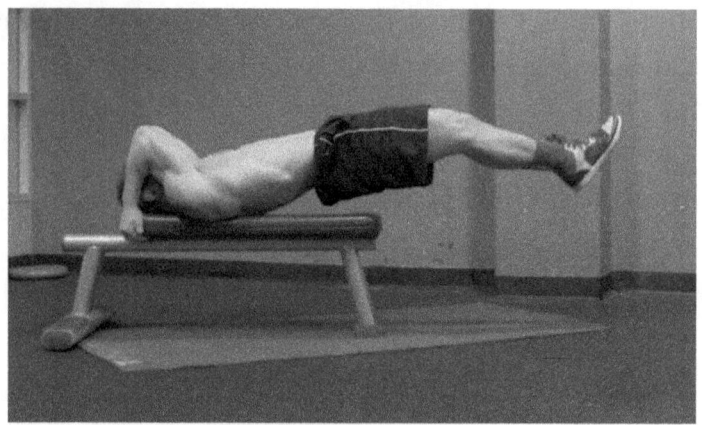

This move was invented by Bruce Lee, and is a very tricky maneuver to execute, therefore, you should only attempt it after you have been exercising for a while and gained some core strength. Form is also very important if you want to avoid injury, so ensure that when you are doing this exercise you leave no weight on your vertebrae.

To begin, lie down on your back on a bench, or the floor, ensuring that you have something behind your head to grab on to for support. Raise your legs, glutes and lower back into the air, leaving only your head and shoulders on the ground or bench.

While keeping your body in a straight line, and resisting gravity, lower your body back down as slowly as possible. Once you feel the need to increase the challenge, do not allow your legs to touch the ground, but lift them back up just before to increase the work your core is doing.

45. Side Lunges

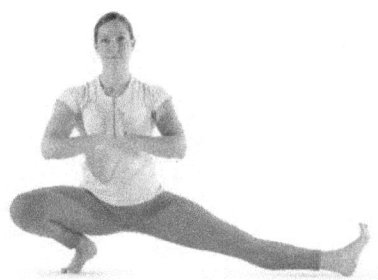

Stand up straight, with knees and hips slightly bent. Your feet should be shoulder-width apart. Keep your head and chest up. Start with this position. Take a small step to the right and keep your toes pointed outwards. Slide your left leg and extend your left knee while you push your body weight to the right. Hold this position. Change the legs after a few seconds.

46. Crossover Lunges

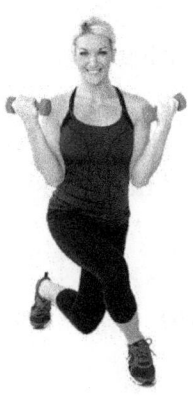

Get to the starting position of a basic lunge. Cross your left leg over the right leg and try to lunge as far as you can to the right side as you land on your heel. Change the legs over to do the other side. This can be easier if you do it with a walking forward motion.

47. Alternating Plyometric Lunge

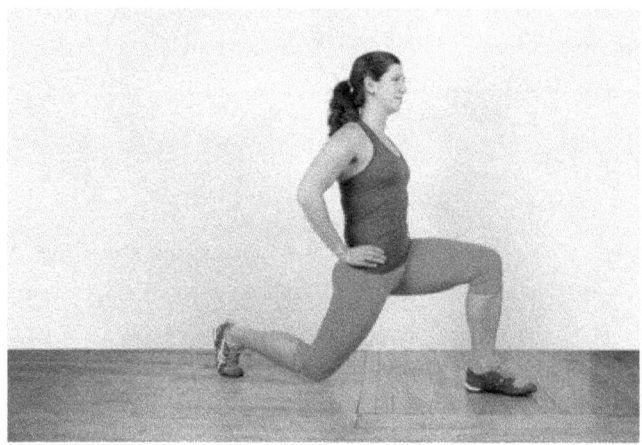

This is a great exercise to work on your quads and groin, and also build your glutes and hamstrings. Begin by standing up with your feet shoulder width apart. Then, once you are in a complete lunge and your knee is close to the ground, jump back with force and change your leg positions while you are in the air.

When you land, return to the lunge position. Repeat this several times to create a set. Remember to keep your arms straight and rigid and balled into fists.

48. Walking Lunges

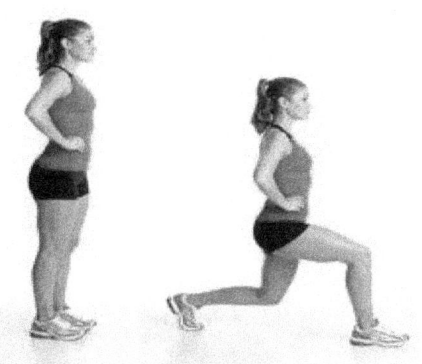

This exercise begins with you standing up straight with your hands on your hips. Step forward and lower your hips as if you are doing a standard lunge, however, instead of moving back to the original starting position when you are coming back up, move your back foot forward so that you end up ahead of where you started. Repeat the process for the opposing foot.

49. Reverse Lunge with Front Kick

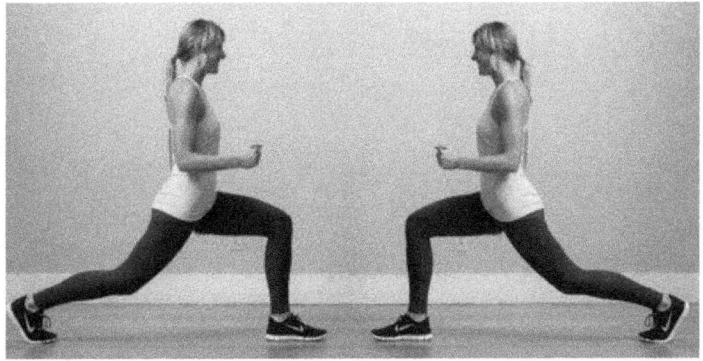

Begin by standing upright with your feet a shoulder width apart. Take one step back and then bend your knees until you are in the lunge position, keeping your arms up and bent at the elbow. Launch into a front kick, by extending the foot that is bent behind you upwards and kick as high as you can. Go back into start position and repeat with the other leg.

50. Jumping Lunge

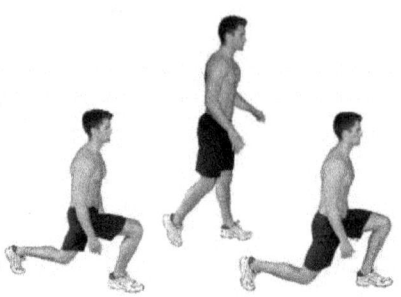

Start this exercise by standing up straight and tall, and from this position, into a lunge. After the lunge, push yourself off from your feet and the bottom and jump. While you are in the jump switch up your legs and then land and return into the lunge position.

51. Corkscrew Lunge

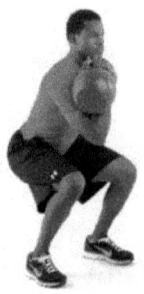

This exercise is a great way to work out your abs and your lower body at the same time. To perform a Corkscrew Lunge, stand up straight with your hands behind your head and perform an ordinary lunge by placing your right foot in front of you and lowering your hips until both of your knees are at a 90° angle with the ground.

While you are doing this, twist your upper body, bringing your left elbow towards your right knee. Return to the starting position, and repeat the lunge again, this time changing the leading leg.

I hope you have learned something from this book so far and would greatly appreciate it if you could leave an honest review on Amazon.com.

Workouts for Abdomen

There are some good exercises for your abdomen and you can follow them to burn the fat of your love handles and tummy.

52. Warrior Poses 2

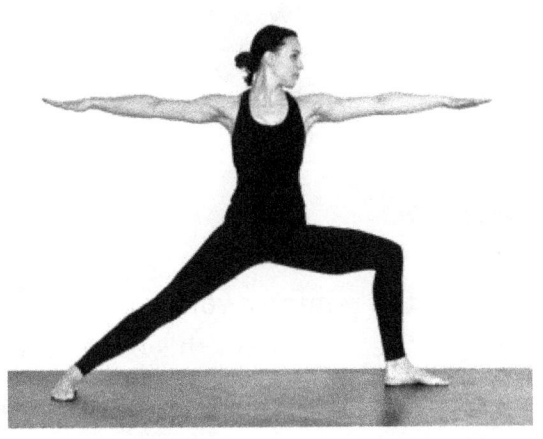

The posture is good to increase the strength of your muscles, thighs, abdomen, and back. It is an effective posture to lose weight.

It is quite similar to Veerbhadrasana, but there is a little difference. There is no need to raise your hands above your head because you have to raise hands on the either sides. Extend your fingers and keep them parallel to your right and left leg.

Turn your head to see in the same direction of your right hand. You can repeat this posture to get maximum benefits. The posture is not for you if you are suffering from diarrhea and high blood pressure.

53. Chair Poses

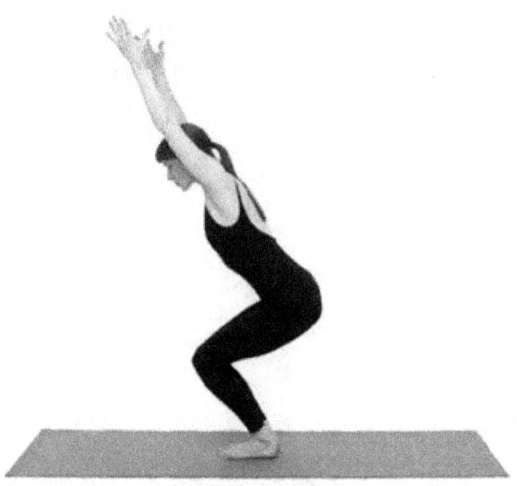

The posture is perfect to reinforce your core muscles, tone your buttocks and thighs. Steps to follow this posture:

Stand straight on the calisthenics mat and join your hands in front of you. Raise the hands above your head and bend your knees to have a parallel direction on the floor.

Twist your torso in the forward direction and deep breath. You can stay in this position as per your capacity, and gently move back to the standing position to avoid any injury. The posture is not good for those suffering from knee or back injury.

54. Tree Pose

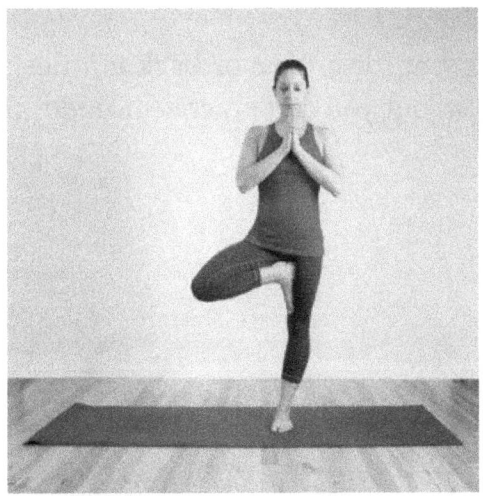

The posture is great to tone the thighs and arms and abdominal muscles.

Stand on your legs by joining them and exert your major weight on one leg and a little weight on the other leg. Lift your leg on which you have less weight toward your opposite knee while keeping your foot in the inward direction.

Hold your ankle to give support to your leg while pulling up. Lay your heel of the foot on the inner thigh of the other leg and keep it as close to the pelvis as possible. Now softly raise your both hands above your head while pointing your fingers toward ceiling.

It is important to maintain your balance and keep the focus of your mind on your posture. Breathe constantly and have your focus on one spot to balance your posture to avoid falling over. There is no need to take the support of the chair while doing this posture because it will decrease the intensity of the posture.

If you are suffering from knee or back injuries, the posture is not good for you, but you can practice it under the supervision of an expert.

55. Squats

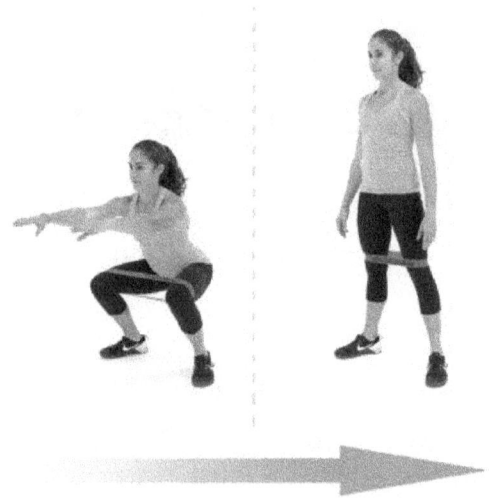

These are usually beneficial for legs and trains primarily the muscles of the thighs, hips, and buttocks. Stand with feet a little wider than shoulder-width apart. Hips stacked over knees and knees over ankles.

Keep the head facing forward with eyes straight ahead for a neutral spine. While the butt starts to stick out, make sure the back stays straight, and the chest and shoulders stay upright.

56. Burpees / Squat Thrust

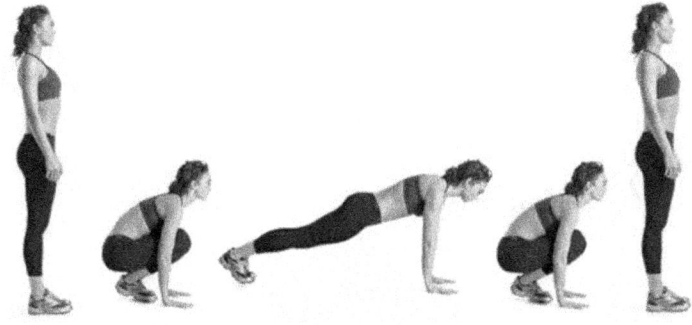

Burpees are a full body exercise which virtually works a lot of muscles in the body, from abs, glutes, & hip flexors to chest and shoulders. You can burn more calories in a lot less time.

The start position is, standing straight with your feet shoulder-width apart and hands by your sides. Squat down and place your hand's palms down on the floor in front of your feet.

Jump up your legs out behind you until they are fully extended. Do one full push up and jump your feet forward to just behind your hands. Use an explosive motion to push through your heels and return to the start position.

57. Explosive Jumping Lunges

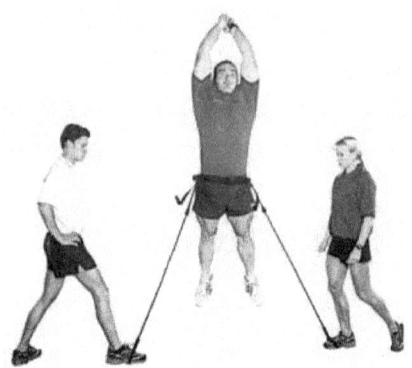

Targeting primary muscle groups: Quads and Hamstrings.

Secondary: Abs, Calves, Glutes & Hip Flexors.

Stand straight with a tight core and your chest up. Lunge forward with your right leg then put your hands on your hips and jump up. Switch your leg midair and land with your left leg in a forward lunge. Alternate sides for one minute.

58. Hanging Leg Raise

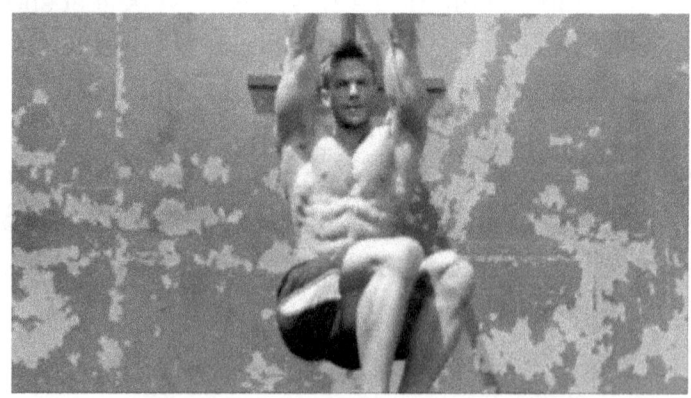

The hanging leg raise is a core strengthening exercise that targets the entire abdominal area and improves stability in the lower back and helps strengthen other muscle groups such as your arms, shoulders and even your legs.

Grip a pull up bar with a firm overhand grip. Raise your legs until the torso makes a 90-degree angle, then lower your legs slowly until they are straight and repeat.

59. Ab Exercises

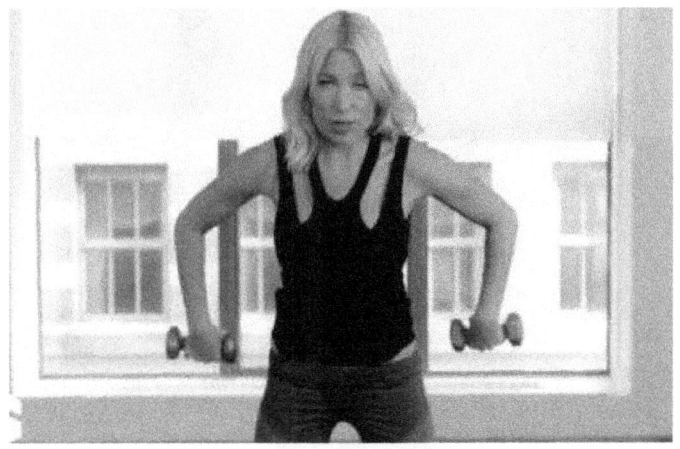

Abdominal area workouts help you get more control over your body movements besides giving you appealing six-pack abs.

There are several benefits associated with ab exercises. For example, it helps your body to attain a better posture because your muscles will be stronger. Also, those workouts will banish back pain, and you'll notice that your lower back will be more flexible, and your digestion will improve through regular stomach exercise as well.

If you're starting an exercise routing to decrease your excess fat, it's important to focus on the lower abs first because this area is the most difficult to strength and tone. The upper abs will tone and tighten naturally as the lower abs become stronger.

60. Jumping Jacks

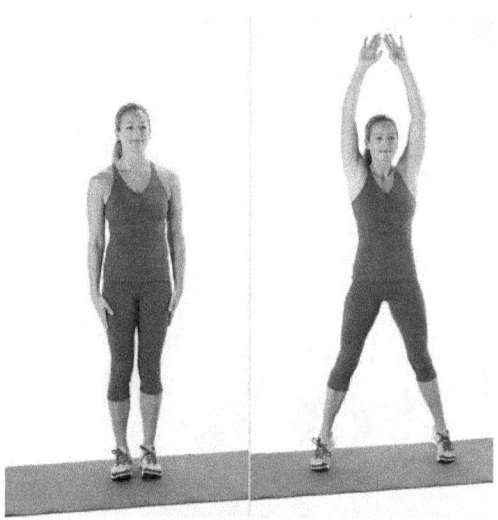

Do you remember doing jumping jacks during gym class at school? If you were like me, you hated them and did not think they worked any muscles. It felt as though the only thing they accomplished was warming you up. You may have felt hot and sweaty afterword with no real accomplishment made.

Jumping jacks are a callisthenic and they do indeed work out your muscles. They also burn calories and fat away. Jumping jacks encourage you to take in more oxygen as you jump, as you breathe deeply and quicker as you jump.

To do a jumping jack, stand up straight and be sure that there is nothing too close to you or you could injure yourself by hitting it. Jump up and bring your arms together over your head, palms touching. Your feet will be side by side when you land. Jump again and swing your arms and legs out in an "x" shape. Your arms will be above your head. This is one jumping jack.

Remember, proper form and quality is more important than rushing through the exercise and trying to rack up a quantity. Do not rush through the exercise. This could cause injury and can cause the exercise to not be effective. Maintain proper form and you will be rewarded with toned muscles.

61. Bicyclers

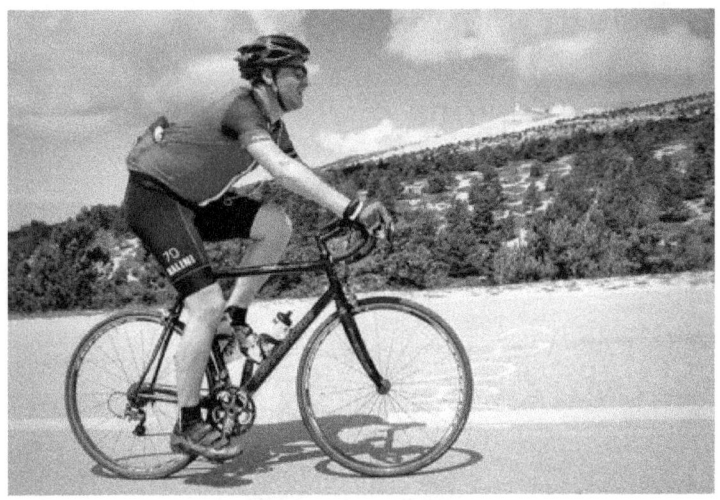

The bicycler exercise is kind of like a crunch or a sit up. It works out your abdominal and back muscles.

To do a bicycler, lie on the floor. Press your lower back onto the ground. Put your hands behind your head and weave your fingers together loosely. Create a forty-five-degree angle by lifting your knees. Move your legs as if you were peddling a bicycle. When you extend your right leg, bring your right elbow to meet your left knee. When you extend your left leg, bring your left elbow to meet your right knee. Keep your core engaged during this exercise.

Do not use your arms and hands to hold up your head. Do not pull the head up and strain the neck. Keep your elbows back and don't let them migrate forward.

Remember, proper form and quality is more important than rushing through the exercise and trying to rack up a quantity. Do not rush through the exercise. This could cause injury and can cause the exercise to not be effective. Maintain proper form and you will be rewarded with toned muscles.

62. Hyperextensions

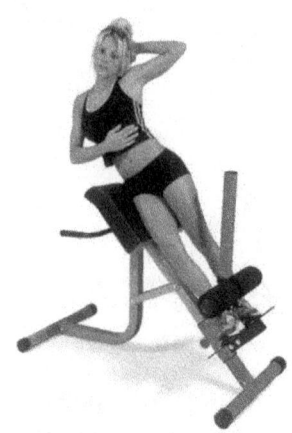

Hyperextension? Isn't that an injury you can get to your knee when you step too far forward? No, in fact, this is not a medical term at all. It is a fun, easy callisthenic you can do anywhere, even in bed.

To do a hyperextension, you will need to lie down on your belly. Lie straight with your arms by your sides. When you are ready, lift your feet, head, and arms up as far as you can. Your shoulders will be back and your will try to lift your chest off the ground.

Engage your core and your glutes as you do this exercise. Gently place your body back on the mat with your head to the side until you are ready for the second repetition. Hold for as long as possible each time. As you practice more and more, you will be able to raise your entire chest off the ground.

In another variation of this exercise, you can reach your arms out in front of you or over your head.

Remember, proper form and quality is more important than rushing through the exercise and trying to rack up a quantity. Do not rush through the exercise. This could cause injury and can cause the exercise to not be effective. Maintain proper form and you will be rewarded with toned muscles.

63. Ski Jumps

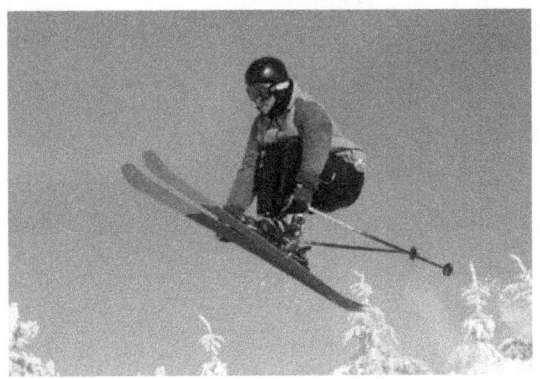

Ski jumps are an exercise that, unlike their name suggests, you do not have to be out in the cold for!

To do a ski jump, stand with your legs hip-width apart. Put your shoulders back and your arms back as if you were holding on to ski poles. Bend as if you were skiing and jump from side to side. You can use a line or rope as a guide. Land with your legs hip width apart. This can be a fun, easy way to burn calories and gain endurance.

Remember, proper form and quality is more important than rushing through the exercise and trying to rack up a quantity. Do not rush through the exercise. This could cause injury and can cause the exercise to not be effective. Maintain proper form and you will be rewarded with toned muscles.

64. Mule Kicks

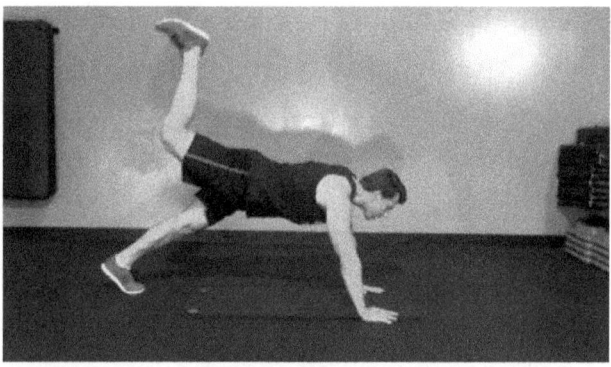

Also called donkey kicks, mule kicks shape your glutes and your core.

To do a mule kick, start with your hands and knees on the ground. Engage your abdominals, drawing them to your core.

Extend one leg until it is parallel to the floor. Draw it back to the starting position, then extend the other. Keep your back straight and do not let your shoulders drop, as this can cause unnecessary strain on your muscles and tendons. Keep your neck straight as well.

Remember, proper form and quality is more important than rushing through the exercise and trying to rack up a quantity. Do not rush through the exercise. This could cause injury and can cause the exercise to not be effective. Maintain proper form and you will be rewarded with toned muscles.

65. Flutter Kicks

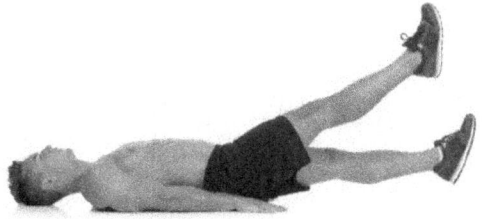

Another type of kick, flutter kicks work your abdominals, especially your lower abs, and your hip flexors.

To do a flutter kick, lay flat on the ground. Keep your shoulders on the floor. Lift up your legs. Kick one leg up quickly, then return to hover over the floor. As you return it, simultaneously kick the other leg up next, then return to hover over the floor. Keep your back and your legs straight. Do not kick up too high.

Remember, proper form and quality is more important than rushing through the exercise and trying to rack up a quantity. Do not rush through the exercise. This could cause injury and can cause the exercise to not be effective. Maintain proper form and you will be rewarded with toned muscles.

66. Jogging

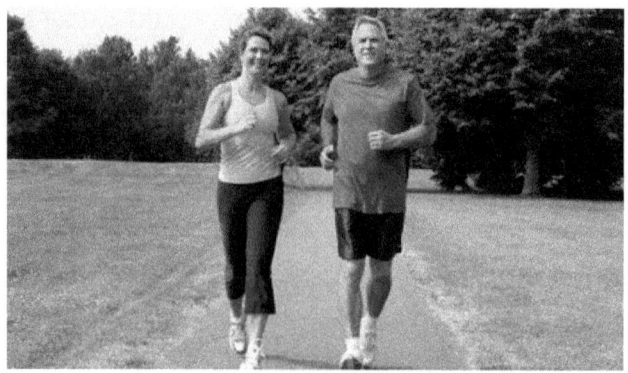

You may not do much running now that you are an adult, but maybe you did when you were young. Jogging can make you feel free and is a great way to enjoy fresh air and nature. Jogging is an amazing way to lose weight and gain muscle. It tones your legs and core.

To jog, you will need some jogging shoes. There are the two different types of shoes. Traditional jogging shoes have a 10-12 millimeter drop between the heel and toe of the shoe. The drop is the height of the shoe from between heel to toe. These shoes also offer heel cushioning. The other type of shoe is a barefoot shoe. These shoes have zero drop between the heel and toe.

Find a trail to jog on that is well-traveled. If you plan on running when it may be dark, such as early morning or evening, you will also want a paved trail and a well-lit trail. Start off slow. Alternate walking and jogging as you work up to the speed, intensity, and incline you want.

Remember, proper form and quality is more important than rushing through the exercise and trying to rack up a quantity. Do not rush through the exercise. This could cause injury and can cause the exercise to not be effective. Maintain proper form and you will be rewarded with toned muscles.

67. Swimmers

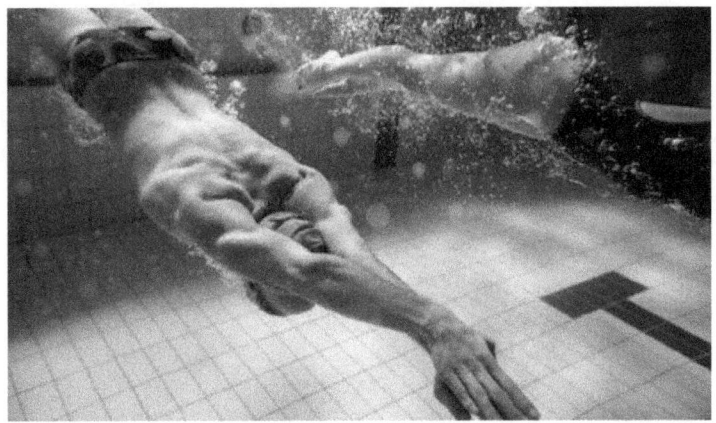

Do you like swimming? Do you wish you could swim on land? With this swimmer's exercise, you will be exercising your muscles like you would be if you were swimming.

To do a swimmer's exercise, lay on your belly on the floor. Stretch out your arms and legs. Lift your right arm and your left leg higher than your opposing limbs, like you were paddling as you swim. Keep your core engaged. As you drop these limbs, raise the others.

Swimmers exercise works the abdominal muscles, the glute muscles, and the hamstrings.

Remember, proper form and quality is more important than rushing through the exercise and trying to rack up a quantity. Do not rush through the exercise. This could cause injury and can cause the exercise to not be effective. Maintain proper form and you will be rewarded with toned muscles.

68. Jump Rope

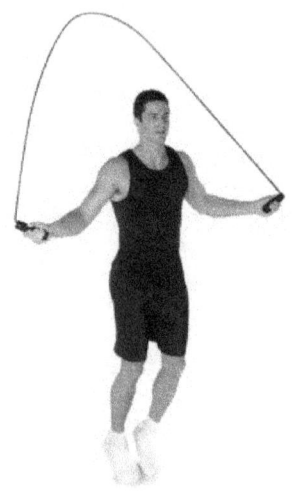

Do you remember jumping rope to this rhyme? You may have jumped rope to this or many other rhymes when you were young. Did you know that jumping rope is a fun, easy way to lose weight? Did you know that jumping rope is also a callisthenic?

Jumping rope is an easy callisthenic to add to your workout. To jump rope, you will need a jump rope. You can jump rope barefoot or wearing shoes. Start with the rope behind you.

Using your wrists, circle the rope up and over your head. When it reaches your feet, jump! Continue jumping as it circles around over and over again. Now you're jump roping!

Jumping rope can also be done socially. You will need two other friends to swing the rope and you can either start standing in the middle or you can jump in. You can even use two jump ropes.

This is called Double Dutch and is fun and harder than using only one rope. Jumping in and out of the ropes takes concentration, but is rewarding. Jumping rope can help you build endurance and stamina.

Remember, proper form and quality is more important than rushing through the exercise and trying to rack up a quantity. Do not rush through the exercise. This could cause injury and can cause the exercise to not be effective. Maintain proper form and you will be rewarded with toned muscles.

Don't forget to share your thoughts on this book by leaving a review on Amazon.com It takes just a few seconds.

69. Crisscrosses

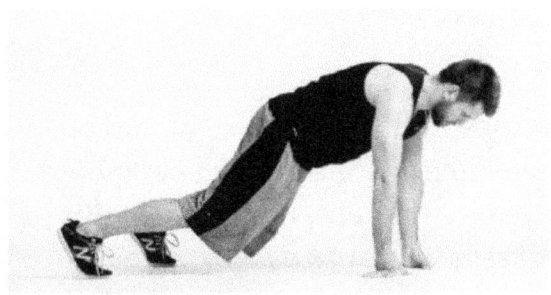

This exercise is good for toning stubborn areas of flab in the legs. In order to do a crisscross, get down on your back as if you are about to do a rep of sit-ups, just like you would for sit-ups put your hands behind your head.

Now just raise your legs up in the air and start crossing your legs in midair while you do a kind of twisting sit-up with your torso, pulling your neck and stretching your abdomen.

Repeat these crisscrosses as many times as you can within your 3-5-minute time frame. This is a great way to strengthen your legs and tone the rest of your body. It's just a simple crisscross but it does a lot when it comes to shaping those more stubborn areas of flab.

70. Full Body Roll Ups

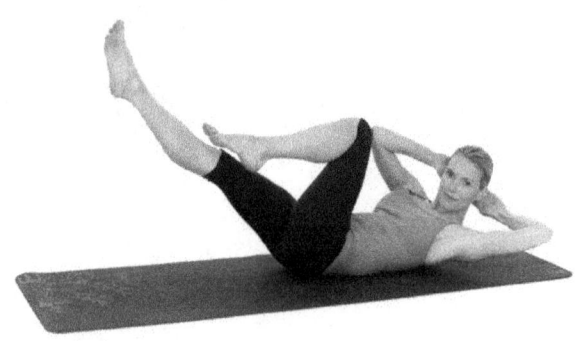

In order to do these roll ups, you need to start off by laying down flat and then holding your hands high over your head. This will help you to exercise your abs. Freeze frame this pose as long as you can and then curl your arms back to you.

Just a few of these roll ups will really serve to build upon your routine. It's just a matter of just rolling yourself up at full length and then unfurling back at equal speed. A full body roll up is also quite a full body work out.

71. Side Plank Push Ups

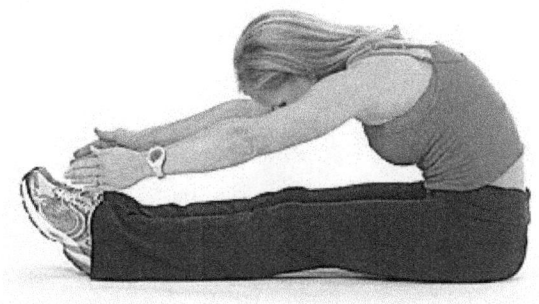

This is a rather fun callisthenic exercise that anyone can do. Start out on your knees with your hands under your shoulders, making sure to keep your core parallel to your legs. Finally, bend your arms and try to keep them I place while you drop your chest to the ground.

Basically, stretched out to your full length with one hand on the ground and propped up on your side, you can do a pushup with just one hand.

This exercise will quickly build muscle mass and is a great way to build upon your callisthenic progression routine. So, make like a plank guys and do those side push-ups!

72. Monster Squats

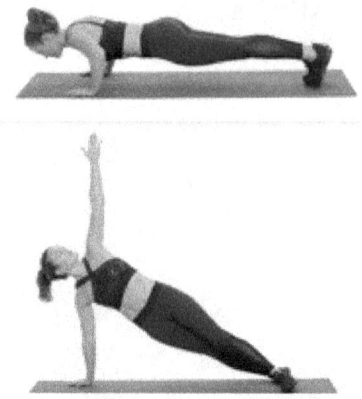

This callisthenic exercise builds upon the regular squat in a really big way. And these monstrous squats can work to help you with your thigh, glutes and calves like none other!

To do this one, simply stand with your right and left foot apart from each other at shoulder width, keep your toes pointing forward and try to keep your arms right in front of you as if you are about to start sleepwalking! Now just rise up!

Keep rising up like this and you will soon be burning fat and building muscle! You should do this exercise as many times as you can within a 3-5-minute interval. It doesn't take much time to get a really monster of a result.

73. Pistol Squats

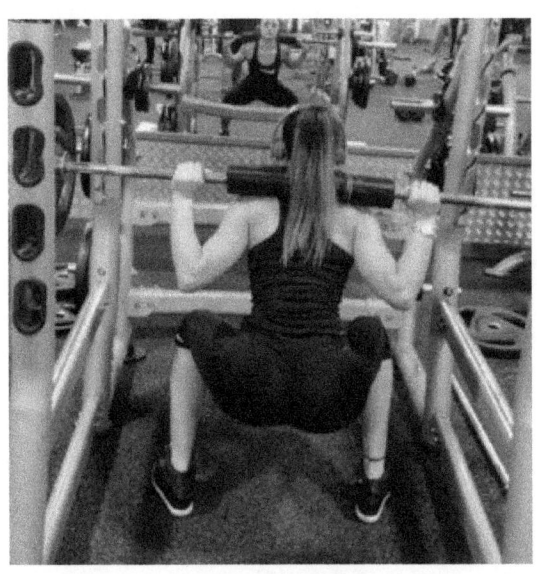

This is a great callisthenic progression for toning up your leg muscles. Basically, just keep your balance with one leg in the air, and then from this one-legged standing position slowly squat down to the floor.

Now rise back up and feel that burn! This exercise greatly benefits the muscles of your thighs, calves and glutes like no other!

Definitely make Pistol Squats a part of your circuit and callisthenic workout routine! This exercise may be a little bit more difficult than others when you first try it out, but after you build up a bit of strength and endurance things will begin to run very smoothly.

Much more than improving the tone of your lower physique, this exercise also has some athletic benefit, helping to improve balance and ability. Give it a try!

74. Mountain Climb

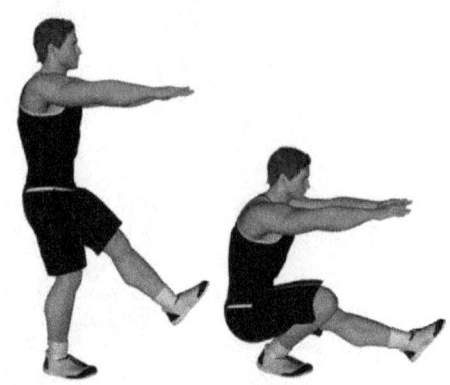

As the name of this workout might imply, for this one you need to position yourself as if you are climbing some sort of obstacle. This primes you for the symbolic and literal climb you are undertaking in your fitness routine.

In the climbing pose, begin moving your knees up to your chest in quick, rapid movements as if you are racing up the mountainside. Keep your back pointed toward the ceiling the whole time, and be sure to alternate your legs as you progress.

This exercise progression expels a lot of energy and as a result burns up a lot of fat. As well as feeling the calorie and fat burn however, you can also get a real workout for your heart, giving your cardiovascular system a nice and steady boost.

Just as the physical act of climbing real tangible mountains can get your body in great shape, even the climbing of these imaginary callisthenic mountains can get your body nice and trim too! Climbing mountains can bring some great benefit!

75. Inverted Rows

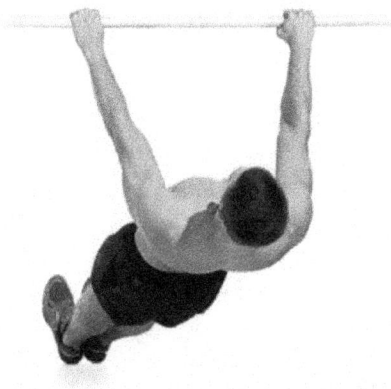

They are perfect for developing your arms to be thick and strong. They also help improve your posture and your upper back

Start by positioning a bar in a rack which should be about your waist line. Get into your starting position by taking a grip which is wider than your shoulder width on the bar as you hang underneath the bar. At this time, your body should be straight as your heels rest on the ground while your arms are fully extended.

Start by flexing your elbow to pull your chest up towards the bar. Your shoulders should be drawn back when you are doing this movement. Once up, pause for a moment and then return back to the starting position. Repeat the whole process for 2 sets of 6-8 reps each.

76. Pull-ups

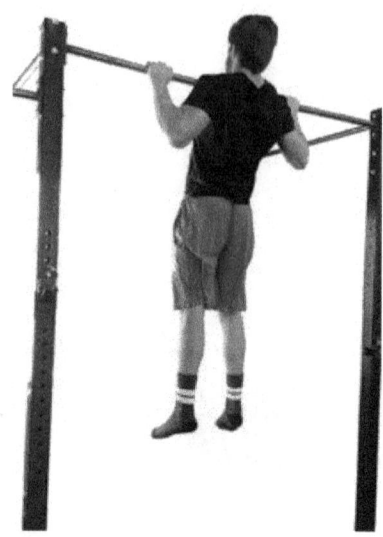

This is a great way of starting your calisthenics exercises. Pull-ups are good for building your upper body strength. This exercise works your anterior, triceps and pectorals.

Start by setting up a pull-up bar then grab onto the bar about shoulder- width with palms facing down. Now raise your feet by bending your knees and hang on to that pull-up bar with straight arms.

The next step is for you to pull yourself up past your elbows and way up until your chin surpasses the pull-up bar. Then lower yourself down until your arms are straight. Take a breath and pull yourself up again.

Did You Know You Are MOST Likely Burning Fat Too SLOW?

Discover The Most POWERFUL Method to Start Burning Fat Up to 400% Faster!

For this month only, you can get Bruce's best-selling & most popular book absolutely free – *The Most Powerful Method to Burn Fat Up to 400% Faster!*

Get Your FREE Copy Here:

TopFitnessAdvice.com/Download

Discover exactly what you need to do to **put your metabolism into hyperdrive** and have your **fat melt away effortlessly**. And learn the biological "hacks" that have been scientifically proven to **boost the rate that your body burns fat by up to 400%.** With this book, readers were able to reach their fitness goals significantly quicker, so it's highly recommended that you get this book, especially while it's free!

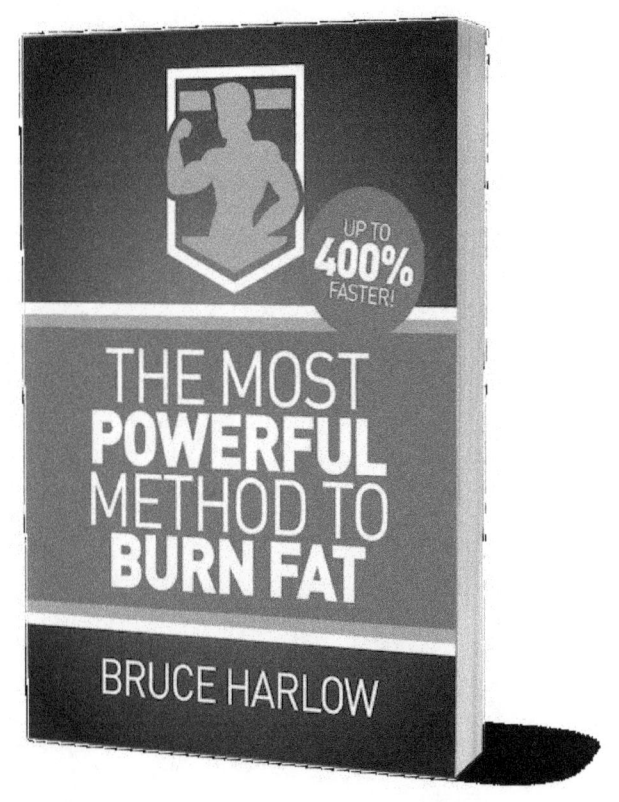

Get Your FREE Copy Here:

TopFitnessAdvice.com/Download

Conclusion

A noteworthy misstep that beginners tend to practice, by way and large, is that they won't take after or play out the activities as they ought to be finished. Thus, their outcomes are miniscule, best case scenario and following a couple of months of diligent work, and they basically give up after.

Keep away from this no matter what by perusing through the activities we have drilled down completely and tailing them EXACTLY as the headings say to do. You will never have the capacity to develop the solid muscles that you need the length of you don't do the activities accurately.

Moreover, recollect to warm up before you do the activities. You never need to neglect to warm up before you do the activities. The reason for warming up and extending is to warm up your muscles and get your heart rate going. In the event that you don't warm up and extend before a work out, you're requesting inconvenience.

We're not saying that you ought to wear yourself out with extending, yet we are stating that you completely need to get your muscles warm and your heart rate raised. As it were, work up only a little sweat before you work out for the huge sweat.

As a last expression of guidance, recall to be understanding and perceive that it requires investment to get comes about. Step by step begin with less sets and reiterations for the less exceptional activities first.

At that point, steadily increment those quantities of sets and reiterations before moving up to the more exceptional activities. On the off chance that one particular piece of your body feels frail, concentrating on practicing that some portion of your body with another work out. In a couple short months, you will begin to see the outcomes that you've for some time been imagining about.

Final Words

I would like to thank you for purchasing my book and I hope I have been able to help you and educate you on something new.

If you have enjoyed this book and would like to share your positive thoughts, could you please take 30 seconds of your time to go back and give me a review on my Amazon book page.

I greatly appreciate seeing these reviews because it helps me share my hard work.

You can leave me a review on Amazon.com.

Again, thank you and I wish you all the best!

Enjoying this book?

Check out our other best sellers!

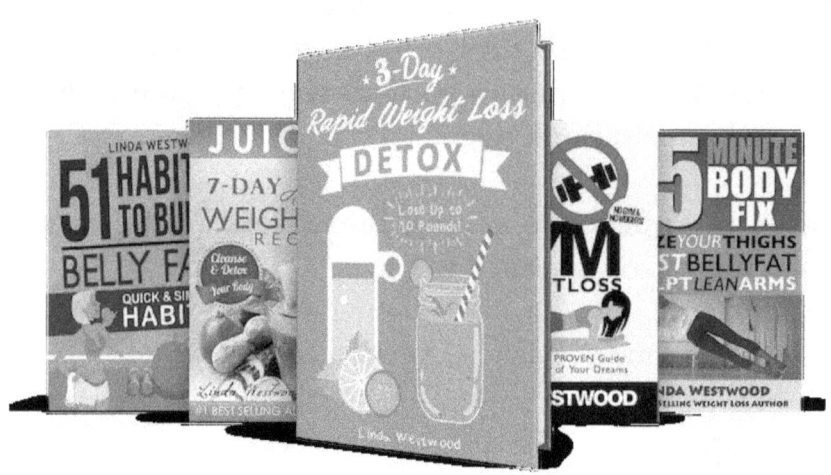

Get your next book on sale here:

TopFitnessAdvice.com/go/books

www.ingramcontent.com/pod-product-compliance
Lightning Source LLC
Chambersburg PA
CBHW031200020426
42333CB00013B/764